"It's a miracle!! You cannot believe the freedom that comes when you're following the program. After years of living in the hell you describe (that most of us have experienced), it seems impossible that there is something that takes that hell away. I am having a very hard time understanding why after years of suffering, I'm waking up feeling good, motivated, silly, happy. I'm beginning to be the person I really am. It's crazy but true! I feel like taking the message to the mountaintops! But life is strange; one only stumbles upon such a miracle when one is ready to hear. So many people need to hear this."

—*Anon*

"I was so impressed with the message which was so RIGHT for my husband and me, that I went immediately to the Internet site and contacted K.D. to set up sessions with her during our recent trip to America. We drove from California to Albuquerque to see her and were blown away with her radiance, clarity and message! It WORKS! Our lives have begun the process of transformation to radiance. Thank you Kathleen . . . you have changed my life forever!"

—*S. A., Geneva*

"I just want to thank Dr. DesMaisons for breaking me free of my sugar bingeing cycle. For years I ate self-destructively, eating, hating myself for eating, and then eating again because I hated myself, and so on. Then my mom told me about the book—she has lost 20 pounds without any trouble! This sugar sensitivity information and simple program has changed my life. I no longer feel the constant gnawing hunger and have been able to take control of my eating and from there my self-esteem. I have lost 12 pounds and am feeling better than ever. Just in time for my wedding, too!!"

—*E. B., Ithaca, NY*

"For the first time in my life I am not fighting constant hunger. I always knew we had alcoholic relatives, and my mother was hypoglycemic, but until I read your book I never correlated the two. It makes perfect sense! In the past seven months I've lost 20 pounds effortlessly. I enjoy exercising but the weight NEVER came off, not before this program. I've recommended your book to my daughter and my niece and each has lost 12–15 pounds. Thanks for your good work."

—*A., Redwood City, CA*

"I read *PNP* in May and have been following the principles ever since. I have lost a total of 28 pounds without feeling deprived. I am no longer on depression medication and feel plenty of energy. I just want to thank you for all your research and personal investment that resulted in this book that has helped so many people. I am so grateful that there indeed is something I can do to help myself."

—*A., Corvallis, OR*

"Immediately pinpointed myself in numerous areas of your book. Have successfully attended weddings, funerals, and parties without NEEDING any sweets. My self-esteem is coming back—I have tackled two part-time jobs and have interviewed for a new full-time one. Just two months ago I was curled up in my chair fuming over what a failure in life I was (the first month or so was rough while my body adjusted). I still have a ways to go yet, but being able to wake up in the morning—and the first thoughts NOT being suicidal—is definitely a big boom. Your book has done for me in four months what my general practitioner and my homeopathic practitioner couldn't do in three years."

—S. M. T.

"I'm in my third year of recovery and THIS year is the worst rollercoaster of trying to balance my protein/sugar/mood swings. Was at wit's end, wondering where could I find a doctor who knew addiction recovery AND nutrition when my sis sent me a blurb on your book. Went to bookstore and the words leapt off the cover at me! I KNEW it was more than just blood sugar; I had been doing food combining, protein in the a.m., etc., for years, even before I quit drinking. You have saved my life and more important, my peace of mind, by filling in the blank spaces in my diet management. All I want is to feel normal after I eat! Even after I had the blood sugar thing down, I was still experiencing weird feelings, and there they were in the book: a column for beta-endorphin and one for serotonin! Thank you so much for giving me direction!! God bless you! I have been telling everyone about your book."

—M. S.

"You saved my life! The book filled in the blanks I had tried in vain to do for twenty years of nutritional studying before and especially after I quit drinking! Thank God! Now I have a good orderly direction to take! I'm NOT going crazy or losing my mind. Thank you so much, love the website."

—M. S., *Ponte Vedra Beach, FL*

"Thanks Kathleen for your concern and your efforts to produce *Potatoes Not Prozac*. I know I'm sugar sensitive and sugar addicted. I'm looking for the courage to let go of sugar and the emotional and physical "rewards" I think (feel) I'm getting from it. Books like yours and the website help the message sink in. I was moved to tears by a letter I read in your review section . . . this does run in families . . . it was signed by my beautiful sister hundreds of miles away from me and in the same pain. Thanks again for your great SEVEN STEPS!"

—P. N., *Atlanta, GA*

"I am hypoglycemic. For how long, I don't know—perhaps all my life. It took me a long time to figure this out! As a child growing up I was SO overweight. I just ate all the wrong foods. My mom was wonderful. She just didn't know. They took me to lots of doctors. THEY didn't know. I'm so happy for your book and for your web page. This is especially important, I feel, for alcoholics and children of alcoholics, who are often in this category. THANK YOU! Please send copies of your book to physicians."

—B. G.

"I'm wondering, could this all possibly be true? I am seven years in recovery from alcohol, five months in recovery from nicotine addiction, but still struggling with years and years of food issues. I just knew that it was more than willpower or lack of knowledge. I have read nearly every book written on food, dieting, nutrition, compulsive overeating, etc., and tried just as many diets/food plans but this was the first book that made sense to me."

—L. H.

"I always knew I used food as a drug but never understood it. I am a recovering alcoholic and long before my drinking I had food problems. I was always starving myself and no matter how thin I was I felt crazy. Now eight years into recovery I am just starting to understand the entire disease process and how food has always been part of it. I am working the steps in order now and just adding the protein and using a carb at night has been so helpful. Thanks."

—K., Antiga, WI

"Kathleen, you have my gratitude, respect and admiration! During the first four years of my sobriety from drugs and alcohol I gained over 60 pounds, telling myself that "at least it wasn't vodka" when I would microwave a nightly pint of Häagen Dazs, or have a huge bowl of pasta for breakfast on weekends. Now, six years and one child later, I have a commitment to both physical and emotional health and vigor—and the strong desire to see Nicholas reach his own adult-hood without his mother constantly weeping, being couch-bound, or dead."

—T., Tucson, AZ

POTATOES

not

PROZAC

Updated Edition

Kathleen DesMaisons, Ph.D.

POCKET
BOOKS

LONDON • SYDNEY • NEW YORK • TORONTO

First published in Great Britain by Simon & Schuster UK Ltd, 1999
First published in the USA by Simon & Schuster Inc. 1998
This updated edition published by Pocket Books, 2008
An imprint of Simon & Schuster UK Ltd
A CBS COMPANY

Book design by Nancy Singer

3 5 7 9 10 8 6 4

Simon & Schuster UK Ltd
1st Floor
222 Gray's Inn Road
London WC1X 8HB

www.simonandschuster.co.uk

Simon & Schuster Australia
Sydney

A CIP catalogue record for this book is available
from the British Library.

ISBN-13: 978-1-84739-053-0

Printed and Bound in Great Britain by
CPI Cox & Wyman, Reading, Berkshire

The recommendations in this book are not intended to replace or conflict with
advice given to you by your doctor or other health care professional. If you have
any pre-existing medical or psychological conditions, or if you are currently
taking medication, you should consult with your doctor before adopting the
suggestions and procedures in this book. Following these dietary suggestions may
impact the effect of certain types of medication. Any changes in your dosage
should be made in cooperation with your prescribing doctor.

This edition of *Potatoes Not Prozac*
is dedicated to the countless people
whose fierce desire to heal lead us all
to deeper knowing of a solution
that changes lives.

CONTENTS

ACKNOWLEDGMENTS

The revision of *Potatoes Not Prozac* is a testament to the more than half a million letters and email I have received from men and women all over the world. People from every state in the USA, Canada, Mexico, the United Kingdom, Ireland, Sweden, Denmark, Germany, France, Italy, Croatia, Crete, Turkey, Iran, Japan, Argentina, Australia, and New Zealand have been talking with me.

These voices have refined the original vision. These lived stories spoke to the power of the seven steps. This edition includes those voices, and includes revisions and upgrades directly related to what we have learned together in the last ten years.

I am deeply indebted to everything our community members have offered to building a broader story.

This dialogue has been made possible by a group of men and women who serve the community by acting as volunteer leaders. Our leadership team is skilled, dedicated, and unswerving in their commitment. I offer my humble thanks for their time, energy, and recovery. They made the vision come alive.

POTATOES
not
PROZAC

INTRODUCTION TO THE
NEW EDITION

Before you delve into this second edition of *Potatoes Not Prozac*, I want to give you some background on our program for healing sugar sensitivity. It helps to have context when making a decision to trust a healing program. How can you know whether this program works? Is this just one more promise that will turn to dust over time or is there really something to it? To answer those questions, let's connect with the power of both the science behind the methods and the lived experience of those who are doing the *Potatoes Not Prozac* program.

THE SCIENCE

Science is an exciting tool in helping you understand how your body works. Countless men and women working in academia around the world are asking questions and seeking new answers: They develop careful experiments to test a hypothesis. Then they publish their experimental results in peer-reviewed journals to invite critique and confirmation by their peers. The process is rigorous and demands careful scrutiny on one question at a time.

The strength of this process comes with the scientific dialogue over years of validation. A major constraint of this process *is* that it takes years to evolve and also depends upon funding that may be affected by a changing political climate. Even more problematic is that science books are about data rather than real people who are living complex, messy lives. Scientists work to exclude the complexity and contradiction of messiness by focusing on one variable at a time, attempting to exclude what are called "confounding variables."

Field clinicians work directly with people rather than simply manipulate numbers. Clinicians are in the trenches of everyday life.

When I started the process of looking at the science, I was a clinician in the field of addiction. I brought years of experience to the table. I had worked in mental health, nutrition, and public policy. I had started and run an addiction treatment center and had listened to thousands and thousands of clients. This professional experience, added to the personal background I will tell you about in chapter 1, motivated me to find more answers in science.

My educational training was nontraditional and interdisciplinary. Rather than enter a field, I wanted to create one. Rather than narrow my scholarly work to one question, I wanted to find answers to the questions that arose in my work with people. So I came to the scientific literature from an outside-the-box perspective and started reading in many fields. I read the literature for addiction, psychology, nutrition, and neuroscience. Here are the facts I gathered and began writing about in the first edition of this book.

- The brains of alcoholics are different from other brains. This special configuration is inherited.
- There are people who are sensitive to carbohydrates and have a more powerful blood sugar response to eating them.
- When needed, the brain releases opioids (natural painkilling chemicals), and these can affect your choices of what you eat.

- Sugar acts like an opioid drug, such as morphine and heroin, in the brain.
- The kind of foods you eat and the timing of your eating can affect your mood.

All these facts had been established in the scientific literature by 1996, but the very nature of scientific research (which looks at one thing at a time) meant that the people doing the alcohol studies were not looking at the nutrition findings, and the nutrition folks were not thinking about the connection to genetics. For example, the questions being explored about sugar as a drug were along the lines of "Can we use sugar as a painkiller in infant circumcision?"

Because my clinical experience was based on listening to people's experiences—which did not divide themselves neatly into discrete scientific categories—I was able to conceptualize a theory that crossed all the relevant disciplines. My working hypothesis was:

- There is an inherited biochemical condition called *sugar sensitivity* that has predictable and specific effects on the brain and on a person's behavior. The foods a sugar-sensitive person eats and when they eat them will affect them profoundly.
- Sugar has the same painkilling and euphoria-stimulating effect in the human body as opioid drugs do. These drug effects of sugar are heightened in sugar-sensitive people. Sugar addiction, like drug addiction, is real and can open the gate to other addictions.
- Changing what sugar-sensitive people eat and when they eat it can have a profound effect on their well-being and behavior.

Using this working model, I wrote *Potatoes Not Prozac*, which (despite the title) was really about healing sugar sensitivity. Since the book's publication in 1998, there have been more developments in the field as science continued asking questions and finding answers. Early in 2000, Bart Hoebel, a senior researcher at Princeton University, heard about the hypothesis I had developed on sugar sensitivity and decided to test it in his laboratory. In 2002, Hoebel and an undergraduate student, Carlo Colantuoni, published a paper confirming sugar addiction in rats, titled "Evidence that intermittent, excessive sugar intake causes endogenous opioid dependence." In 2005, Cyrilla Wideman published the results of a study demonstrating that the effects of sugar addiction, sugar withdrawal, and sugar relapse are similar to drug addiction, withdrawal, and relapse (the article was entitled "Implications of an animal model of sugar addiction, withdrawal and relapse for human health"). Not only was the term sugar addiction being published in peer-reviewed scientific journals, but reference was now being made to sugar addiction in humans.

While science was catching up, the first edition of *Potatoes Not Prozac* offered people a way to understand what was going on with their sugar-sensitive bodies and heal themselves. People found the book and started to connect with me and with each other on my Radiant Recovery® website. The heartwarming success I had seen with the alcoholics in my clinic was now happening with sugar addicts, binge eaters, yo-yo dieters, people with eating disorders, and people dealing with depression and a multitude of other diagnoses. These people were hugely comforted to discover that their sugar addiction was real. Just as when Alcoholics Anonymous redefined alcoholism as a disease, when I explained that sugar addiction is caused by a chemical imbalance, not a character defect, sugar-sensitive people were suddenly free of societal (and self-) condemnation. But there was more to the story than just the science of it.

THE EXPERIENCE

The lived experience of people doing the program revealed to me a kind of code to behavioral change that I could then embed in the steps. The seven steps of the program are not just about changing your food (such as eating sufficient protein at each meal), they are about participating in a *process* that converts addictive behaviors into recovery skills. You *will* heal your unbalanced, sugar-sensitive brain by following the program, but you will do much, much more. You will heal your addictive behavior and begin a life of radiant recovery.

Being born sugar sensitive means that pretty early on you get wacky. Even as a child, you can start being moody, impulsive, mouthy, withdrawn, stubborn, dramatic, or reactive. As your diet stays off-kilter, these early responses set in as behavior patterns. People think this is your personality. You buy into this, and as you grow older the behaviors expand to include all-or-nothing thinking, self-absorption, grandiosity, helplessness, and a deep feeling of being "less than," despite outward appearances. You develop the Dr. Jekyll/Mr. Hyde dichotomy that I will talk about in chapter 1.

Doing the steps of *Potatoes Not Prozac* slowly, in order, and as outlined creates a process that makes for deep behavioral change as well as dietary change. The steps are infused with a "miracle drug" called recovery. You learn to listen, to yourself as well as to others. You learn to wait, to have patience, to plan, and to go slowly—all of which may be anathema to you now. You learn to see the consequences of your choices, you make connections between what you eat and what you feel. You learn to ask for help, let others guide you. You move out of isolation and find that you are not the only one with this problem and that change is possible. What you thought was your personality is not who you are at all. It was a result of your sugar-sensitive biochemistry, your imbalance, and your old way of eating.

Each of the seven steps builds on the one before it. The process is developmental. You are never given more than you can do based on the biochemical healing that is happening. As you do the steps, the process heals you. Your "personality" shifts and the best of sugar sensitivity (yes, there is a good part) emerges. You enjoy being smart, intuitive, compassionate, tenacious, funny, thoughtful, and skilled. You become someone you really like. And the other shoe does not drop. Life simply gets better and better.

The wonderful thing is that you do not have to work on all these behaviors individually. You do not have to master your blood sugar and your serotonin and your beta-endorphin, you just "do the food." When you do the food, your body and your process take care of the rest.

There is a part of you that has sensed this truth all along. It is why you respond so deeply to the content of the books I write. This new edition of *Potatoes Not Prozac* is more specific in its recommendations, and it has been expanded to reflect ten more years of experience with sugar-sensitive people doing the program. We are no longer cutting a new trail—now you have a superhighway clearly marked to get you home!

DR. JEKYLL AND MR. HYDE

Are you aware of your *self*, smart, and sensitive to others' feelings? Are you committed to your own personal growth? Do you care about things deeply? Do your friends value you and respect your opinion? Are you successful in your work? Are you usually confident and hopeful about your future?

But do you sometimes also feel your confidence slip away, leaving you in self-doubt and despair? Does it seem "crazy" that you can be so clear one day and so desperate the next? Worse, you may drop from the heights to the depths in the same day. It's almost as if there were another person inside of you.

You hate to admit it, but you can be moody and impulsive. You want to get things done, but your attention drifts. You lose energy and get tired. You crave sugar and turn to sweets and snack foods to get yourself going again. Sometimes you eat compulsively. You put on weight. You seem to have no self-discipline. You often feel depressed and overwhelmed.

You may have consulted your doctor. You may have gotten counseling from your pastor or a psychotherapist. You may have been put on Prozac or one of the other antidepressants. Maybe things got a little better for a while. But something is still wrong. Your life is still not the way you want it to be and you can't seem to find an answer that works.

If this description fits you, you may be sugar sensitive. Your body chemistry may respond to sugars and certain carbohydrates (such as bread, crackers, cereal, and pasta) differently than other people's bodies do. This biochemical difference can have a huge effect on your moods and your behavior. How you feel is *physiologically* linked to what you eat—and when you eat it.

Listen to Emily's story.

I was overweight, depressed, and exhausted all the time. I had a lot to be grateful for in my life, but something was wrong. Why didn't I feel better about myself? Why was my battle with those extra twenty pounds so hopeless? Why didn't I have the energy to do more in life? I was so discouraged.

I drank several cups of coffee a day, snacked on gummy bears, and ate healthy foods like pasta, vegetables, and fruits. I avoided fats and high-calorie desserts. Sometimes I grazed throughout the day, sometimes I'd skip meals and eat only once a day. Although I had tried lots of diets, I always regained the weight I lost. I would start an exercise program, stick to it for a few weeks, then go off my diet and stop exercising. I still was overweight and hating it. I felt like a failure in this part of my life and I was ashamed of it.

Often I couldn't sleep and I was plagued by anxious feelings. Sometimes my heart would start racing for no reason. I had sudden outbursts of crying or anger. I tried therapy, figuring I was just "not right." But it wasn't enough.

So I went to my doctor and told her my long list of problems. She looked concerned and ordered a series of exams. I, too, was concerned. Maybe I was starting menopause early. I even worried I might have a brain tumor. A week later my doctor called. "I have good news and bad news," she told me. "The good news is that you are not in menopause and you don't have a brain tumor. The bad news is that I don't know what is happening. Your lab tests and your physical exam results are all normal."

Frustrated and depressed, Emily came into my private practice in Addictive Nutrition. She told me she was a recovering alcoholic with nine years of successful sobriety and had heard that I was using nutrition to help people with her symptoms. After listening to her story and asking her some questions about her background and her eating habits, I recognized what was wrong. I had seen it time and again in women and men who came through the door seeking help for compulsive eating, alcoholism, drug addiction, or the same strange cluster of symptoms Emily had—symptoms that had not responded to other treatments.

Emily was neither clinically depressed nor suffering from the effects of a bad childhood. She was not weak-willed or lazy. She was sugar sensitive. Emily had inherited a special kind of body chemistry that made her more vulnerable to the mood-altering effects of sweet foods and refined-flour products than her friends. She was caught in a vicious cycle of emotional highs and lows controlled by her blood sugar levels and her brain chemistry. Emily's body responded to sugar as if it were a drug.

SUGAR SENSITIVITY

Sugar sensitivity turns a person into Dr. Jekyll and Mr. Hyde. It's like having two different people live in your body. From one moment to the next, your fine sensitivity and openness turn into moodiness and irritability. Your confidence and creativity dry up, only to be replaced by low self-esteem and hopelessness. Your vision for the future dissipates into the frustration born of not following through.

This emotional Ping-Pong remains inexplicable without an understanding of sugar sensitivity. Like Emily, millions of people who have inherited sugar-sensitive bodies are caught in the pain of not understanding a problem that controls their lives. Sugar-sensitive people seem to know instinctively that something is wrong but cannot make sense of what it is.

Do you feel this way? If so, your intuition may be right on target. If you are sugar sensitive, you are not inherently weak-willed or without self-discipline. Your behavior reflects a skewed body chemistry, which you have tried to correct unconsciously by self-medicating with sugars and simple carbohydrates.

Your sugar sensitivity is a problem you inherited. You did not create this dilemma. It is not your fault. What's more, it is a problem that can be solved. I have an answer that you have been seeking for a long time. Clear and simple, the solution to sugar sensitivity makes perfect sense. As you begin to understand how your blood sugar levels and brain chemicals work and how they interact, you will start to appreciate the power of your own body. Instead of being driven by your body chemistry, you will begin to chart your own life. You will find a straightforward explanation for the behavior you have struggled with for so long—and a straightforward solution based on giving your body the kinds of foods it needs to keep your emotions in balance and your life in forward gear.

This book tells the story of sugar sensitivity and how to find the radiance that comes with having your biochemistry in balance and at your service.

NAMING THE PROBLEM

The story of sugar sensitivity comes out of my own personal history and my work with thousands of clients in addiction treatment. After a long career in public health, I started an addiction treatment center in 1988. I wanted to make a difference in people's lives. The typical recovery rate for alcoholism was—and is—

dismally low. People who had treatment relapsed. And they relapsed again—and again and again. Although addiction experts had tried many alternatives, the picture remained pretty grim. A 25 percent success rate was considered good. But accepting the fact that I would not be able to help three out of every four people who came into my clinic was out of the question for me. I knew there had to be a better way, and I set out to find it.

My determination to beat the odds comes out of my personal history. When I was sixteen, my father died of alcoholism at the age of fifty-one. He was a brilliant, sensitive man who couldn't find his way out of the bottle. They say he loved to party as a young man; by the time he reached middle age he was drinking a fifth of vodka every day.

My father stayed sober for one year, the year I turned eleven. He was a career officer in the U.S. Air Force and his superiors had threatened to discharge him from the service if he didn't stop drinking. So he went into detox and rehabilitation for the first—and only—time. I remember that year well. With my father sober, life was so much better for all of us. Everything I had secretly dreamed of was happening and we finally lived like a normal family.

One year later, despite being sober, my father was discharged from the air force for alcoholism. Past job evaluations had followed him and the air force did not recognize—or perhaps did not believe—his commitment to sobriety. In losing his job, my father was cut from his lifeline. His sobriety and our family's newfound stability careened rapidly downhill. Five years later he was dead.

It took me twenty-five years to grieve the loss of my father. At the time I felt only relief—relief that I no longer had to be ashamed of his drinking. All I wanted then was a normal teenage life. After Dad's death, we all colluded in creating a family myth that my father had died suddenly of pancreatitis. In reality, he had been dying of alcoholism for five years, but not one of us ever talked about it. We just carried on, folding our wounds into the tapestry of our lives, each trying to make sense of the tragedy alone.

"Don't Tell, Don't Feel, Don't Share"

My history has shaped me deeply. Because of my father's alcoholic behavior I learned to pay close attention to the interpersonal dynamics around me. I learned to immediately "read" the emotional temperature of almost any situation. I learned to grow up early, become a high achiever, be the hero in my family. Most of all, I learned the inviolable rules of an alcoholic family:

"What you see isn't really happening."

"Everything is fine, even though you feel something else."

"Don't tell. Don't feel. Don't share."

I learned to live in dissonance. I kept confronting the discrepancy between what the folks around me said was true and what I experienced in my body and in my heart. I challenged my mother about the lies of our family life. I challenged my religious teachers about the difference between what the church said and how people acted. I constantly asked questions about the gap between the ideal and the real. I studied everything I could to try to find a solution for the dilemma of this discrepancy. I wanted to live what I believed and I wanted the world to do the same.

At nineteen, still dreaming of the perfect family, I married and had three babies in rapid succession. But the gap between my ideal life and my real life still loomed large; although smart and successful both in school and as a new parent, I was overweight and subject to extreme mood swings and sudden drops in energy. Sometimes I was filled with self-confidence and felt clear and focused. At other times, I would drift into a sort of "la-la land" and forget to buy milk for the children. My husband thought he'd married Dr. Jekyll and ended up getting Ms. Hyde too. He wondered how my behavior could change so quickly. As for me, I didn't really notice my own behavior. I was well trained to overlook dysfunction, including my own.

My marriage stopped working when my youngest child was six months old. Neither my young husband nor I understood how to make a relationship work and neither of us knew how to ask for help. Single again, I returned to college, worked full-time, and threw myself into the task of raising my children. In the evening, after I had put everyone to bed, I sat on the couch with Coke and popcorn, reading philosophy and folding laundry.

When I was twenty-six, I came down with mononucleosis, which damaged my liver. Because my liver was impaired, alcohol made me sick, so I stopped drinking. It was a straightforward decision, but it probably saved my life. As with most children of alcoholics, I was a sitting duck for alcoholism. My body chemistry was primed to need alcohol, and had I kept drinking I would have gone from enjoyment to dependence to abuse.

Turning to Sugar for Solace

But abstinence from alcohol nudged me onto a different path of addiction. Alcohol hadn't hooked me, but sugar, ice cream, pasta, bread, and soda did. These seemingly harmless foods wrapped me in a cocoon so thick and numbing that I never missed the alcohol.

When I finished college I went on to complete a master's degree in management and counseling. High-achieving child of an alcoholic that I was, I was hired as the director of a nonprofit program before I even finished my degree. Eighteen months later, I was promoted to supervise a hundred staff members. On the outside I appeared successful, competent, and skilled. On the inside I was running from my own feelings. I sensed a huge pool of pain swirling below the bravado of my life. I wasn't aware of the impact of my father's alcoholism on me and I hadn't a clue about what was driving my life.

Finally, at the age of thirty, I could no longer ignore my pain. I realized I needed help and I went into therapy. Because I was the head of a community mental health center, I thought I should maintain the appearance of being emotionally "together." So I traveled four hours and two hundred miles every week to see my therapist. She encouraged me to express my anger. "I won't," I would say. "Anger kills. It isn't safe." For a whole year we argued.

Finally I let myself go and got angry. But my anger was directed not at my father or my family—it was directed at my therapist. I was angry about the direction of my therapy and the dissonance I felt between what she was saying and what she was doing. Two days later she committed suicide. It was hard for me to understand that her death was not my fault. I was just thirty and no one even knew I had been in therapy. "Don't tell, don't feel, and don't share" still drove my response to pain.

I didn't have the skills to make sense of the pain so I turned to doughnuts, a new town, and a new job. Perhaps a new life would make things better. I moved to a place near the ocean. I was comforted by the sea. I lived next door to an ice cream parlor. I was comforted by the ice cream. I gained more weight. The early pattern my ex-husband had identified continued: I was still Dr. Jekyll and Ms. Hyde. When I was good I was very, very good, and when I wasn't, I fell apart. I tried hard to hold it all together, but when I hit forty, I realized that my life would unravel if I didn't find a way to face my pain. The old gap between my inner feelings and my external life had stretched to the limit.

My solution then was to move to California, where the softness of the hills, the sound of the sea, and the openness of the people all soothed me. I reconnected to the child within me who loved to swim and dance and laugh. I started feeling good about myself, but my weight and my mood swings continued to plague me. After every diet I gained back the weight I'd lost. Because I thought my problem with food had its roots in emotional wounding, I worked on my inner development for years. I read hundreds of books, attended dozens of groups and seminars, and filled countless journals with poetry.

No matter how much inner work I did, though, I seemed to be fighting a losing battle. The needle on my bathroom scale was now nearing 240, but I thought the problem was just a matter of willpower. When I developed enough discipline, everything would be fine. As time went on and things didn't change, I lived with deeper and deeper feelings of inadequacy.

Lessons from the "Drunks"

In spite of—or perhaps because of—an inner sense of hopeless-ness, I continued to be committed to helping others heal. I was asked by the county I worked in to start a treatment center for alcoholics and drug addicts. The idea of doing this work felt like "coming home" and I leapt at the chance. Once the clinic got going I found myself frequently abandoning my desk to work directly with our clients. The alcoholics who came into our clinic mirrored both my father's story and my own. They were trying to keep their lives from crumbling beneath them.

Although I had spent twenty years working in public health, I only really began to "get it" about alcoholism and drug addiction when I heard these people's halting voices and listened to their painful stories. What I learned was that what we were doing—counseling, support groups, and pleas for abstinence—didn't work particularly well. Even "good" treatment done by sensitive, car-ing, and trained professionals didn't help much. Our clients kept relapsing despite their best intentions to "work the program." Our recovery rate was no better than the national average. I needed to find out why.

The more I listened to the "drunks," the more I was struck by some missing link between what I heard them say and what I felt. I knew in my heart that their addiction to alcohol was not about a lack of willpower. I knew drinking wasn't an easy way out, a way to escape their unpleasant feelings. Something else was going on. I was convinced that if I discovered this missing link, our treat-ment program for alcoholism might actually succeed.

At the same time, there was a troubling discrepancy between my work at the clinic and my own life. I hadn't used alcohol in eighteen years; I had never formally been in any kind of recov-ery program. I didn't see my compulsive use of food, particularly sugars and carbohydrates, as an addiction. I just thought being fat was a function of my early childhood issues: a thousand failed diets had convinced me that I was a slug who couldn't get it right.

Since I was successful on the outside, I hid my feelings of despair and put in even longer hours.

Yet as I worked with alcoholics and drug addicts, I started to be drawn subtly into recovery. I didn't have a name for my story then, but I began to see that I was going to have to live the principles I was teaching. I didn't want to just teach recovery, I wanted to have it.

This meant I had to confront my past. So I started learning what it meant to be the child of an alcoholic, what it meant to be codependent, and how playing the role of the hero—taking responsibility for others' needs instead of my own—had shaped my professional development. My ending up in charge of an alcoholism treatment center, surrounded by a "bunch of drunks," was no accident. By the grace of something much bigger than myself, I stayed with the process—working on myself while I worked with the men and women at my clinic.

Discovering Food as Pharmacy

My recovery focused on the Twelve Steps that originated in Alcoholics Anonymous, which emphasized surrender to a "higher power." The idea of surrendering to a higher power didn't work for me, but surrendering to something "deeper" did. So I handed my life over to the something deeper and asked for help. One day, by chance, I heard from a friend that she had been doing a food plan that had really worked for her. She was eating protein and vegetables. I tried it. I started losing weight, which surprised and pleased me. But even more astounding was what happened to my cravings and my moods and my behavior. I didn't crave sweet things. I didn't dream about bread and pasta. My emotional ups and downs evened out. I wasn't confused or foggy at certain times in the day. I was able to think clearly. I got things done. I set goals and moved toward them without a constant struggle to stay focused.

Although I had done a lot of work on my inner self, I knew the changes I was experiencing were not psychological. They were *physiological*. I hadn't suddenly gotten my act together. Something had happened in my brain, in my body, and it felt like the missing link I'd been searching for. I had changed my food—mostly by cutting down on sugar and starches—and subsequently experienced a huge change in my physical and emotional well-being. I began to wonder whether, being the child of an alcoholic, I had inherited an alcoholic's body chemistry. Perhaps alcoholics and compulsive eaters like me were hypersensitive to sugar. Perhaps my body physiologically craved sugar the same way my father's body had physiologically craved alcohol. If so, I thought, wouldn't this hold true for my addict clients as well?

So I went to my clients. Asking these men and women what kinds of foods they ate revealed data that were no surprise to me. My clients' eating habits closely resembled my own previous eating patterns. No wonder I felt such an affiliation with these "drunks"! Almost none of them ate breakfast, few ate regular meals, most ate a very high percentage of white bread, pasta, and cereal, and all ate a great many sweets. Whenever I talked to clients who had not been able to stay sober, I found they were eating primarily sweet things and refined-flour products.

Almost immediately I added nutritional awareness as one of my clinic's steps to recovery. I put together a food plan for sugar-sensitive people, a plan based on protein, complex carbohydrates (like whole wheat, potatoes with their skins, and brown rice), fruit, and vegetables. The food plan was simple, easy, and affordable. This plan filled in the gaps I had experienced in my friend's program when I had used it myself. I intuitively knew that eating only protein and vegetables wasn't the best alternative—our bodies need more carbohydrates on an ongoing basis than her plan provided. But if I kept the basic concept, added *complex* carbohydrates, and continued to minimize sugars, I was sure the revised food plan would work. I also added an educational component directed at healing the addictive behaviors of my clients.

I told my clients that this food plan was not a diet, but a way of eating for life. I explained to them my theory about sugar sensitivity and how it might be predisposing them to alcoholism. When I told them that sugar could sabotage their recovery from addiction by making them crave alcohol, they sat up and paid attention. Then they tried the food plan—and got remarkable results.

As my clients changed what they ate, their lives began to improve in a number of ways. Compared to other clients we had seen at the clinic, their withdrawal symptoms passed more quickly and gave them less discomfort. Their mood swings mellowed. Their cravings diminished. Their energy increased. They were more enthusiastic and committed to their recovery than ever. People who had never been able to achieve sobriety began getting—and staying—sober.

After I'd used this food plan with several hundred alcoholics and drug addicts, men and women alike, I found we were achieving unusual success. Our track record told me it was time to establish a scientific basis for the changes I saw coming from my food plan. I decided to leave my job and sell my house to start working on my Ph.D.

Finding Out Why It Worked

My doctoral research took me into professional journals and academic textbooks on nutrition, endocrinology, psychopharmacology, and psychiatry as well as addiction. I learned about the wide-ranging effects of blood sugar and the powerful emotional impact of certain brain chemicals, chemicals that can get thrown out of balance by overuse of sugar.

One of these brain chemicals, serotonin, was becoming better known to the public, thanks to the advent of Prozac, a new antidepressant that boosted serotonin levels and brought feelings of optimism, creativity, and peace of mind. To my astonishment, the other brain chemical I was learning about, beta-endorphin, was as crucial to emotional well-being as serotonin, but it was not being discussed outside scientific circles. My reading showed me that beta-endorphin has a direct impact on a person's self-esteem, tolerance for pain (including emotional pain), sense of connectedness to others, and ability to take personal responsibility for action. You'll learn all about this amazing brain chemical later in the book. First I want to tell you how my story turned out.

As I worked on my doctorate, I found that all the biochemical facts I was learning came together with the results I saw at my treatment center to tell an elegant and compelling story. My research confirmed my suspicions—and the name of sugar sensitivity that I had given to the story of what I saw: some people were indeed sugar sensitive and it had a basis in rigorous science. I was amazed that no one was telling the public about it.

For my doctoral dissertation I conducted a study to measure the effect of my food plan on the toughest audience I could find—multiple-offender drunk drivers. These were people (mostly middle-aged men) who had not been able to stay sober despite huge court sanctions and intensive drunk-driving education and counseling. All of them had already gone through an entire forty-hour first-offender program, had paid thousands of dollars in fines and fees, and had now lost their licenses for eighteen months.

I worked with a group of thirty of these "hopeless" alcoholics for four months, and at the end of my outpatient treatment program, 92 percent of them had gotten sober and stayed sober. They weren't drinking anymore. For the first time in their lives they were experiencing recovery. Eighteen months later, I checked back with the original test group I had used in my doctoral study and only a few were back to serious drinking. The rest had maintained their sobriety or significantly reduced their previous level of drinking. These same results continued as the program grew to serve close to two hundred people.

My success with sugar sensitivity went far beyond helping people to stop drinking, however. At the same time I was working with drunk drivers, my private practice was filled with women and men who were overweight or ate compulsively; adult children of alcoholics who felt tired, crazy, and depressed; and former addicts and alcoholics who, though clean and sober, still didn't feel well.

I became known as "the lady of last resort." When people had tried everything and still felt rotten, they came to me. I taught them about how their blood sugar and their brain chemistry worked, and I showed them how to use my food plan. When they tried it, these people experienced the same miraculous shift that my drunk drivers and I had experienced. Not surprisingly, word began to get out. More and more people from across the country called me for help. I promised I would write a book about sugar sensitivity and the crucial role of brain chemistry.

Potatoes Not Prozac is that book. Since its first publication in 1998, hundreds of thousands of copies have been sold, and I have heard from people from all over the world. I have read half a million letters online. The messages are remarkably similar.

"This book changed my life."

"I wept when I read it."

"I saw myself on every page. It felt like you were in my head."

The original insight I had while working with my small group of drunk drivers has now been tested and acclaimed by men, women, and children from Australia to London, from Sweden to Cyprus, and from every state in the U.S.

Potatoes Not Prozac offers a simple program for counteracting the effects of sugar sensitivity and shows you how to make that miraculous shift in your own life. What's more, you will be able to do this without going on another deprivation diet. You will not have to throw away the foods you love. You will not have to make radical changes that drive you crazy.

The seven-step program I will teach you is a gentle, simple process that respects your style and your needs. You will learn how to read your body and design a food plan that works for you. During this process, I will help you understand the "why" of feelings you have never been able to resolve. You will come to understand what you have known intuitively but been unable to name. You will find an answer you have been looking for.

I wrote *Potatoes Not Prozac* for every child of an alcoholic and every man and woman who is tired of looking good on the outside while feeling bad inside. It is for everyone stuck in addiction, depression, low self-esteem, and compulsive behavior. This book is my story and it is your story. It is the story of all of us who have waited so long and tried so hard to get free of those "crazy" feelings and our Dr. Jekyll/Mr. Hyde behaviors.

2

ARE YOU SUGAR SENSITIVE?

By now you are probably wondering if you, too, are sugar sensitive. And if so, how sugar sensitive are you?

There are two ways to determine this, both of which I use with my clients. Some people prefer the informal approach; others like using the checklist later in this chapter. Let's start with an informal way to diagnose sugar sensitivity. When a client comes to see me about compulsive eating, I start by asking a simple question.

> Imagine you come home and go into the kitchen. A plate of warm chocolate chip cookies just out of the oven sits on the counter. Their smell hits you as you walk in. You do not feel hungry. No one else is around. What would you do?

Does this question make you smile? You may think the answer is obvious, but people who are not sugar sensitive respond by saying, "I go check the phone for messages" or "I go upstairs and put on my sweats." Some will stop and think about whether they would eat some cookies. Others will say, with no emotional charge, "Well, I might try one." People who are not sugar sensitive do not have an emotional response to even the *idea* of smelling fresh chocolate chip cookies.

People who *are* sugar sensitive laugh at the cookie question. Their bodies are already responding to the very idea of the cookies. They know they would inhale a cookie—probably more than one, at that! They might eat the whole plateful, even if they were not hungry. For a sugar-sensitive person, hunger is not the driving motivation. What triggers their desire to eat is the smell of the cookies, the anticipation of how the cookies will feel in their mouth, and the warmth and sweetness of the melted chocolate. Even the feeling of having a cookie in their hand will have a powerful association for them. Those cookies mean love, they mean comfort. Those cookies are friends and lovers.

People who are not sugar sensitive think this response to the cookies is strange, perhaps even stupid: "What on earth are you talking about? Why would I eat a cookie if I wasn't hungry?" But people who are sugar sensitive always know exactly what the cookie question means.

I have asked this question of many, many groups. Every time I've received dramatically consistent reactions. While one part of the group will be waiting for the punch line after I ask, "Would you eat a cookie?" all the sugar-sensitive people are laughing. Their bodies are already responding to the image of the plate, full of warm cookies in the kitchen. Try this experiment with your friends and see what kind of response you get.

Here's a second powerful diagnostic question I use:

When you were little and had Rice Krispies for breakfast, did you eat the cereal for its own sake, or did you eat the cereal so you could get to the milk and sugar at the bottom of the bowl?

People who are not sugar sensitive think the milk and sugar at the bottom of the bowl are disgusting. People who *are* sugar sensitive smile. They remember that the real objective was to get to the dregs of milk and sugar. They got high by tilting the cereal bowl into their mouths and tasting the clump of sugar at the bottom.

Your answers to these two questions may simply reinforce what you already know. Some people—perhaps including you—are very attached to sweet things.

There are lots of other ways to get clues to your sugar sensitivity. You might think back to the size of the bag you carried at Halloween. Children who were not sugar sensitive carried those small orange plastic pumpkins. We carried pillowcases. Their candy lasted until Easter. Ours was gone in three days.

DIAGNOSING SUGAR SENSITIVITY

If you are still asking, how can I know for sure if I am sugar sensitive? let's take a look at the core issues associated with sugar sensitivity. Check each of these ten statements that applies to you:

☐ I really like sweet foods.

☐ I eat a lot of sweets.

☐ I am very fond of bread, cereal, popcorn, and/or pasta.

☐ I now have or once had a problem with alcohol or drugs.

☐ One or both of my parents are/were alcoholic.

☐ One or both of my parents are/were especially fond of sugar.

☐ I am overweight and don't seem to be able to easily lose the extra pounds.

☐ I continue to be depressed no matter what I do.

☐ I often find myself overreacting to stress.

☐ I have a history of anger that sometimes surprises even me.

How many boxes did you check? If you checked three or more, you are reading the right book. If you checked all ten, you are in good company. Each of these statements relates to an aspect of sugar sensitivity. Let's go through them one at a time so you can see what your answers may be telling you.

- **I really like sweet foods.**

Answering yes to this question alone indicates sugar sensitivity. If you *really* like sweet foods, you may have an intense physiological response to them. Sugar-sensitive people actually respond to tasting and eating sugar in a way that is more pronounced than other people. A "normal" person will enjoy sweets but can eat half a cookie and leave the rest for tomorrow. A "normal" person doesn't sit through dinner thinking about dessert. A "normal" person does not feel more confident and powerful after eating sweet things.

- **I eat a lot of sweets.**

Sugar-sensitive people are likely to eat a lot of sweets. Even though you feel you shouldn't, you may eat candy, cookies, or ice cream. Dessert may be the most important part of your meal. You may fast from sweet things during the day and then binge at night.

Or you may really love sweet things but choose not to eat them. Lindsay, a tall, slender client of mine, was sugar sensitive. Because she was concerned about calories and fats in her diet, she had stopped eating hot fudge sundaes, candy bars, and the other sweets she usually craved. But even though she had eliminated obvious sugars from her diet, sweet things continued to find their way into her mouth. She ate energy bars for breakfast. She stopped drinking Coke and switched to fruit juice. She also discovered she loved carrot juice. She would have a glass of wine with dinner as a treat to make up for how much she missed her high-calorie splurges.

All these foods contain high amounts of sugar. Lindsay's sugar-sensitive biochemistry was craving sugars and drove her to eat them even without her knowing what she was doing. Her energy bars and many of the other "healthy" low-fat foods she ate were very high in what their labels called "carbohydrates." Sugars come in many forms. People who are sugar sensitive find them. Go to page 152 for a fuller discussion of sugars.

• I am very fond of bread, cereal, popcorn, and/or pasta.

Your body may respond to foods made with white flour as if they were sugars. You may find you feel good soon after eating them but then feel terrible later on. You may love bread. Cereal may be a staple for you. In the evening, you might settle on the couch with a huge bowl of popcorn.

Rank yourself on a scale of 1 to 10 on your attachment to any of these foods. You may be surprised to find that even though you don't eat "sugar," you have a very powerful emotional attachment to bread, pasta, cereal, and/or popcorn. You would kill for French bread. You know where all the homemade pasta is sold. Don't get nervous. It's okay to feel this way. Your attachment to these foods only tells us how powerful your sugar-sensitive biochemistry is.

• I now have or once had a problem with alcohol or drugs.

If you have used alcohol or drugs in an addictive way at some time in your life, it's very likely that you have a body chemistry that responds more intensely to alcohol or drugs than other people. Your attachment to sugars sets you up biochemically for the addictive use of alcohol and even certain drugs.

Even if you are recovering from alcohol or drug addiction, sugar sensitivity can affect how you feel. This accounts for much of the syndrome called the dry drunk. Hair-trigger reactions and impulsive behavior can be caused by what you eat and when you eat it. Many of the unexplained physical and emotional symptoms that people take for granted in addiction recovery, such as irritability, cravings, mood swings, and sleep disturbances, actually result from having a sugar-sensitive body. In addition, feelings of low self-esteem may continue long after they seem rationally warranted. For example, Christine, who got sober five years ago, expected to feel a whole lot happier and healthier than she does. She has a fabulous job, which she loves, has been promoted three times in two years, and makes twenty thousand dollars more a year than she used to. But she still worries that she will be a bag lady in her old age. The problem is that Christine stopped drinking but didn't change her diet to compensate for her sugar-sensitive body. What and when you eat can make you feel terrible or wonderful.

- **One or both of my parents are/were alcoholic.**

If your parents drank to excess or drank in an alcoholic fashion, you may have inherited a specific type of brain-chemical response to alcohol that makes you feel tearful, depressed, and emotionally overwhelmed—or angry and belligerent—when you are "under the influence" of sugar. You can inherit other aspects of sugar sensitivity as well. Your parents may have been sugar sensitive long before they started to drink. Seventy-eight percent of the drunk drivers in the program I ran reported that their fathers were alcoholics and their mothers loved sweets. This combination of an alcoholic father and a sugar-sensitive mother (or vice versa) maximizes the chance that your were born with a sugar-sensitive body.

- **One or both of my parents are/were especially fond of sugar.**

People who are sugar sensitive often grow up in houses where sweets abound. I remember our family ritual of going to the local Dairy Queen on summer evenings. Ice cream not only created a pleasant memory, it carried a whole emotional charge as well. To this day, the memory of the sweet, cold, creamy soft treat evokes a powerful and pleasant response in my body.

As with the question about chocolate chip cookies, nonsugar-sensitive people do not respond in this way. They may report a childhood memory of going to Dairy Queen, but it's a memory with a different emotional content. Their bodies do not remember the feeling of the ice cream in their mouths with the same intensity. Find a nonsugar-sensitive person and ask them what they remember about food from their childhood. Then ask a sugar-sensitive person. I guarantee there will be a big difference in their responses.

- **I am overweight and don't seem to be able to easily lose the extra pounds.**

Sugar-sensitive people often crave carbohydrates. This isn't an emotional craving, but a physiological one caused by the way their body chemistry overreacts to sweets and carbohydrates. They find dieting difficult and often unproductive in the long term. Restricting calories does not result in weight loss as it should. People who are sugar sensitive can eat as little as 800 calories a day, but if those calories are from carbohydrates, they will still gain weight. They may have tried a low-carb diet and initially had success. But over time it is likely that they started feeling restless and uneasy. Then they slip and eat carbohydrates, cannot get back on the diet, and experience a disastrous rebound effect. You know the "yo-yo syndrome" well: lose ten pounds, regain fifteen; lose fifteen, regain twenty.

- **I continue to be depressed no matter what I do.**

Sugar-sensitive people may have a hard time getting mobilized. You may feel frequently sad or apathetic. You may be depressed and crawl through the day with very little energy. For women, the depression may get worse just before menstruation. Often, sugar-sensitive people are miserable in the winter because the decrease in daylight affects their already impaired brain chemicals. You may self-medicate your depression by eating sweet foods, since sweets are one of the few things that make you feel better, albeit temporarily. You may be taking an antidepressant like Prozac, but still have symptoms of depression. If that's the case, you likely have a sugar-sensitivity aspect to your depression that neither you nor your doctor has recognized.

• **I often find myself overreacting to stress.**

Volatile blood sugar levels make sugar-sensitive people edgy and reactive. You may fly off the handle or cry at the drop of a hat. The conflicting feelings you have don't seem to make sense. For example, my client Shirley worked as a senior manager in a governmental agency. She was well thought of, did excellent work, and liked her job. Most of the time she was steady and clear, but at other times, such as when her boss gave her feedback about her work, she would get overwhelmed and want to sit and cry. She was also surprised by the power of her anger, which seemed to bubble up from nowhere. Like Shirley, you may think of yourself as a really nice person—and most of the time you are. But at other times you feel totally out of control. These mood swings may well be due to sugar sensitivity.

• **I have a history of anger that sometimes surprises even me.**

Sugar-sensitive people can have episodes of anger that seem to overtake them without reason. You may feel like Dr. Jekyll and Mr. Hyde. Your dark side stays hidden most of the time, but those people close to you know it's there. Your flash point is low and your impulse brakes don't work. The intensity of your feelings is particularly scary because it just doesn't seem to fit your "real" personality.

Are these patterns beginning to sound familiar? Does the sugar-sensitive profile fit your experience? Sugar-sensitive people often feel comforted by answering the questions listed above. Patterns in their lives that haven't made sense suddenly start fitting together.

Sugar sensitivity is a theory—a working hypothesis—based on my own observation of how my addicted and/or compulsive clients respond to sugars and on my in-depth investigation of the solid scientific research that has been done on carbohydrate sensitivity and on the role of brain chemicals in alcoholism, addiction, and nutrition.

Scientific research since the publication of this book in 1998 has now demonstrated the physiology of sugar addiction and lends strong credence to my original hypothesis of sugar sensitivity. The stories I originally heard from clients in my California practice and now from the Radiant Recovery® community all over the world tell us that my theory is on target and my program really can help you heal your sugar addiction and your biochemical imbalance. Back in the mid-1990s, naming the problem of sugar sensitivity and offering a solution was too important to wait for the approval of scientific authorities. The findings of researchers are only now catching up with my vision of ten years ago. But hundreds of thousands of people have already used the program since it began to heal their sugar sensitivity and step into the world of what we call "radiant recovery."

Before we go any further, I want to stress that there's nothing "bad" about having a sugar-sensitive biochemistry. The more you can defuse the negative messages you have always received about your behavior, the freer you will be to begin this healing process. Remember that there are millions of people just like you—people who know something is wrong, who joke about being "addicted to chocolate," but who rarely talk about what is really going on inside them.

As you explore the power of your own sugar sensitivity, you might want to ask yourself more questions like this. Try not to be judgmental as you answer. Allow yourself the humor of your "addiction." Perhaps you don't outright lie about when or whether you are eating sweets, but do you lie by omission? Do you eat sweets only when no one else is around? Do you put the bag with the goodies inside something else so people can't see what you are carrying? Do you park your car in an out-of-the-way place to chomp your special treat? Do you hide the candy wrappers under the other trash so your spouse won't know what you ate? Do you eat your children's cookies and then say you don't know what happened to them? Do you go to the warehouse stores and buy huge quantities of candy and tell yourself that it's a good buy? Do you know the hours of the Godiva chocolate store?

CAN YOU BE ADDICTED TO SUGAR?

By now the answer to this question should be pretty clear to you. Yes, you can be addicted to sugar, to sweet foods, and to white-flour products that your body responds to as sugars. This addiction is physiological and affects the same biochemical systems in your body that are affected by drugs like morphine and heroin. You can actually get "high" on sugar. Eating it can make you feel euphoric immediately afterward. If you don't have your regular sugar "fix," you may experience withdrawal symptoms. Yes, you can become *physiologically* dependent upon the effect the sugars have on your body.

Being sugar sensitive means you have a special biochemistry. You have a different relationship to sugar than a person with a "normal" biochemistry. Your heart sings at the sight of a newly opened box of candy, your molecules seem to jump to attention when you get a whiff of chocolate. This sensation of your body jumping to attention is not about greed. It is the natural physiological response of a sugar-sensitive person whose brain has just released a powerful chemical called beta-endorphin in response to a certain smell.

When you eat chocolate, is there a part of you that actually feels a greater level of self-esteem? This may seem like an outrageous idea, chocolate enhancing self-esteem. But chocolate releases beta-endorphin, and beta-endorphin causes an increase in feelings of self-esteem. Your relationship to sweet things is operating on a cellular level. It is much more powerful than you have realized.

In my sugar-eating past, I never understood why I felt so much better after I had candy. I knew it was emotionally comforting, but it didn't make sense that I felt so good after doing something so "bad." Sometimes I would binge and start soaring with a sense of possibility about what I could do with my life. I would write plans in my journal, make lists, and feel confident that the world was all right. A few hours later I would crash and feel like nothing good would ever happen for me, no change would ever come; I would end up a bag lady with nothing to show for my life.

It felt crazy. How could I possibly feel such contradictory things—and feel them almost from one minute to the next? I remember the day I sat in the library working on my Ph.D. and first read about the impact of beta-endorphin on self-esteem. The hair on the back of my neck stood up. I suddenly saw the connection. I was eating chocolate as self-medication to achieve self-confidence. Instead of feeling totally stupid about my behavior, I began to see that there was wisdom in it. Consciously I wanted to feel better and more secure, and unconsciously I knew there was a relationship between chocolate and self-confidence. Of course I turned to chocolate when I felt down.

The problem is, sugar-induced self-esteem doesn't last very long. And having your self-esteem wear off that quickly is a pretty fragile way to live. The good news is you can evoke beta-endorphin-linked self-esteem without the negative and addictive effects of chocolate. You do not need chocolate! You need self-esteem based on an inner sense of well-being that comes from biochemical balance, clarity, and feeling healthy. What you eat can have a huge effect on how you feel. I will show you how to develop a food plan that can help you overcome the drawbacks of the sugar-sensitive body you inherited.

You can make sense of what is happening in your body. Learning about sugar sensitivity will give you a perspective that takes away the negative charge you have carried all these years about your eating. You will shift from thinking you have character defects to understanding that you have a body with a volatile blood-sugar response and low levels of beta-endorphin and serotonin. You will understand that your body and brain have a heightened reaction to sweet foods, and that you really can have such a thing as a sugar addiction. You will learn that many of the behaviors that you hate about yourself are simply part of the sugar-sensitivity picture. And you will learn how to change all these things by changing what and when you eat.

The good news about biochemically based behavior is that it *can* change and it can change *fast*. You do not have to pursue years of psychotherapy to get results. You can start making sense of behavior today by learning which foods affect you negatively and why. You can start changing what you eat and feel better right now. You can discover what thousands and thousands have learned and reported to me about the relationship between doing the food plan and the profound changes they have experienced in their lives. Below is the transcript from one of our online chats; this one was with a group of women from the United Kingdom and Sweden. They have been doing the program between six months to five years.

radiantkd	**I would like to talk about how it was "before" and how things have changed. How were they before step one?**
Anna Marie	angry, violent, wild, outta control
Anna Marie	BE [beta-endorphin] spiking cycles all over the place
Marti	heartburn
Shelley	I felt crazy
Chris	totally bonkers
Shelley	anxiety, depression, bingeing

Diane	BS [blood sugar] crashes and some of them I didn't realize
Ivy	I am way too close to the "before" so think I will just listen :-)
Anna Marie	depressed, suicidal, angst
Heidi	oh geez, before step one? I was mental. Tantrums, meltdowns, depression, hopelessness
Lulu	irritable
Nancy	mood swings, exhausted, overwhelmed, lonely
Anna Marie	inappropriate boundaries
Suzanne	done to
Anna Marie	and sharing
Chris	moody, angry, all alone
Diane	I, too, was crazy, depressed, high, bingeing
Heidi	angry, mean, nasty, moody, tired, bored, overwhelmed
Ashley	crazy, madwoman, depression, hopeless, overwhelmed, out of control—I once smashed up the kitchen (red face)
Suzanne	no boundaries at all
Josie	Not understanding and feeling so guilty
Chris	totally helpless
marydenmark	rollercoaster
Diane	oh, yes, afterwards, lots of guilt tripping
Marti	totally codependent but not knowing about the concept
Anna Marie	Wondering if Mr. Hyde was taking over . . .
Josie	Trying so hard to get on top of things
Shelley	gaining weight very fast
Suzanne	soooo tired—wiped out at night
Anna Marie	couldn't focus
Chris	yeah, extremely sleepy
Shelley	yes, Suzanne, no energy—too tired to cook :)
Diane	always trying to "catch up" and "get organized" (actually still not totally there—but feeling ok, baby stepping my way there now ;)

Chris   oh yes!
Suzanne   bingeing on sweets

radiantkd   **all of the above?**

Nancy   Yep—all of the above!
Mannie   Right Kathleen
Heidi   zero concentration
Ashley   too muddled to cook
Ivy   All of the above plus total exhaustion and despair
Heidi   muddled is a good word, Ashley
Anna Marie   foggy thick brain
Shelley   yes, Heidi
marydenmark   never felt like doing anything
Mannie   :D As long as we've said wacko . . . I'm in
Diane   oh, I hate that foggy thick brain : (
Suzanne   Yes Shelley—and never had any food in the house
               or any plans. "What do you mean bod—are you
               hungry again???!"

radiantkd   **and trying to act normal?**

Chris   trying to pretend to be normal
Lulu   or even thinking I was normal :)
Nancy   Always pretending things are normal
Ashley   oh to "the world" I was a high achiever, confident
               and capable hehehe
Shelley   yes, trying to put on a brave face
Heidi   doing a pretty good job on acting normal but then
               bingeing and melting down at night
Diane   wondering why everyone else seemed to be so
               "together" and why I couldn't seem to do that
               at all
Ivy   I think I thought that WAS normal, and every-
               one else just dealt with it better.

Anna Marie	oh yes, showing an "all together" face to everyone
Josie	All or nothing attitude—"tomorrow I'll be different"
Ivy	Oh yes Josie!

radiantkd   **and shame?**

Anna Marie	oh yeah waiting for that magic something to make it all better at once!
Diane	yes, lots of all or nothing—still working on that one . . .
Nancy	Right Josie—tomorrow, next week, next month, I'll. . . .
Marti	still got plenty of that!
Suzanne	yes tomorrow I will start my new life! (yet again!)
Mannie	for not having it together . . . Yes.
Ashley	shame I couldn't control the temper or the drinking
Ivy	That word gives makes my hairs stand up—so much shame.
Chris	bucket loads of the stuff
Shelley	big shame
Josie	And then tomorrow I didn't do it, and then the guilt and feeling so weak and hopeless
Diane	yes, shame, but I always thought of it as guilt—what's the dif?
Anna Marie	shame that I was such a mess and couldn't let it on to anyone or get any help
Suzanne	loads and loads of shame—being diabetic and not being able to quit sugar . . .

radiantkd   **ok, talk about how it is now.**

Heidi	calm
Anna Marie	big

Heidi	peaceful
Chris	happy
Shelley	calm
Anna Marie	facing the past
marydenmark	much more stable

radiantkd	**think about the other side**
Chris	content
Nancy	content
Diane	much more clear, patient with myself most of the time
Penny	steady and happy, understanding
Ashley	calm, steady
Shelley	capable
Ivy	Utter, blissful relief
Anna Marie	seeing patterns
Heidi	patient
Ashley	clear
Suzanne	balance
Chris	bright-eyed and bushy-tailed
Suzanne	patience
Diane	wanting to work things out and learn
Heidi	contented is my best word. just happy being who I am doing what I do.
Nancy	focused
Ashley	joyful
Ivy	full
marydenmark	more like rolling hills
Marti	purposeful—more measured
Ashley	happy
Ivy	controlled
marydenmark	than rollercoaster
Nancy	making progress.
Chris	excited (in a good way)

Suzanne	I really like that expression Chris! :)
Marti	seeing the bigger picture
Heidi	capable
Ashley	not afraid but accepting what will come
Penny	happy, even
Diane	yes, Nancy, making progress—nice!
Ivy	trusting
Ivy	peace
Marti	less reactive
Heidi	even is a good one Penny!
Josie	I still do and feel a lot of the same things, but I perceive myself differently.
Nancy	connected
Shelley	committed
Penny	knowledgeable, really, I'm not a mystery to me
marydenmark	boundaries
Diane	when I am feeling "off" I can look at it more from a distance and try to figure out why I am so off.
Josie	have hope

radiantkd	**when you were back there, could you have imagined this?**
Shelley	not in the least
Chris	no way!
Suzanne	no I could not imagine this.
Nancy	nope
Ashley	no. I only kept going because I had nothing left to try.
Anna Marie	not for myself, no
Marti	I find it hard to accept I have "really" changed, like I will put a hex on it all.
Chris	and even if you'd told me I wouldn't have believed you :)

Ivy	the speed of the change astounds me. guess the molecules latched on as fast as they could!
Suzanne	I didn't know I had it in me.
Diane	no way, kd, not imagine—didn't even know what it was!
Penny	had no idea. Thought it was how I was.
Chris	I know what you mean Linda.
marydenmark	no, I knew I was "just that way"
Nancy	I believed I could not have the mood swings and some of that, but I never dreamed I'd find content[ment], peace, focus.

These are real people, just like you. They have not done therapy or spent money. Many of them have never met one another. But doing the food has changed their lives. As soon as you experience the truth of this for yourself, what has been an overwhelming—and perhaps shameful—mystery in your life will become a fascinating journey of self-exploration.

3

IT'S NOT YOUR FAULT

If I am right, then the "crazy" duality in your life, which I call the Dr. Jekyll/Mr. Hyde syndrome, is a result of sugar sensitivity. You may *feel* crazy, but you are not. The problem is biochemical. It's not your fault.

I am going to walk you through understanding why you feel the way you do and show you the way to heal your biochemistry. As we go, you will hear me speak more about radiance—the name we have given to the remarkable state of being that you will experience as you do the program and change your food. People tell me the results they have gotten are beyond their wildest imagination. What's more, as you make these changes, you will not be alone. The support you have extends far beyond this book, and we are going to stand behind you every step of the way.

If you are sugar sensitive, there are three things in your body chemistry that contribute to the "crazy" feelings:

- the level of sugar in your blood
- the level of the chemical serotonin in your brain
- the level of the chemical beta-endorphin in your brain

An imbalance in the level of any single one of these can bring about striking changes in the way you feel or act. When all three are out of balance, it is almost impossible to isolate which one is making you feel so bad. First we'll look at them one at a time, then I'll explain their combined effect to show you why sugar sensitivity can be such a destructive force in your life.

You may have already heard about the impact of your blood sugar level on your well-being. The effects of low serotonin levels has also been widely talked about in the last few years; books about Prozac and several "food and mood" books have examined the value of raising serotonin levels.

But the powerful role of beta-endorphin—a vital brain chemical that affects your feelings of self-esteem, your cravings for sugar, your capacity to handle painful situations, and your feelings of hope (or despair) about the future—is not even being talked about outside scientific circles.

As you learn how these three biochemical systems interact to create changes in your feelings and your behavior, please don't worry about the changes you will be making to the way you eat. The food plan you will develop to counteract the problem of sugar sensitivity does not require deprivation or self-denial. You'll be able to start on that plan in chapter 6. For now, just be tender with yourself and be attentive. The story I am about to tell you is intriguing. Here's what Carrie has to say about it:

> When I started this program I was in a real panic. I had high blood pressure, which was uncontrollable even with medications—terrible mood swings/rages, a lifetime of depression, and edema so bad my legs were hard from my toes to my hips. I couldn't walk much and, since I was fifty-seven, I was terrified I'd have a stroke or heart attack before I got to Step 7.
>
> I had been promised success (which I never achieved) by so many diet gurus that I knew this program would not work. But others before me said it would, that I should

have faith, that I needed to do the steps one at a time. I didn't believe it, but I did it nonetheless because I had run out of options—I'd already tried every diet around.

I questioned eating carbs and fat. "They" [the people in our online community] said it would be okay. I questioned whether it would work for me. "They" said it would. I questioned every single day for six months. I didn't trust it because I'd been fooled so many times. I was depressed and anxious and angry. But I did it.

I could have saved myself the agony. At Step 3 I started losing the extra weight, and it was gone by Step 6 (plus more). My last blood tests were excellent: I moved from the doctor telling me I needed to go on cholesterol medication to the normal ranges in all categories. I don't get edema anymore and I can walk farther and better than I have in years. I don't get depressed and don't have mood swings. I am more honest with myself and others around me—I can admit to being human—and it's paying off because I'm finding I'm an okay person.

—*Carrie*

THE LEVEL OF SUGAR IN YOUR BLOOD

Your body uses a very simple sugar called glucose as its basic fuel. During digestion, all the carbohydrates you eat are broken down into this simplified form so that it can be used by your cells. Glucose is carried by the blood throughout your body to be transformed into energy by your cells as needed. All your cells, particularly those in your brain, require a steady supply of glucose at all times.

When your body has the optimal level of sugar in the blood to supply your cells, you feel good. When your blood sugar level is too low, your cells don't get the sugar they need, and they start sending out distress signals. These distress signals are the symptoms of low blood sugar, a condition also known as hypoglycemia.

The chart that follows shows the difference between how you feel with optimal blood sugar and low blood sugar:

OPTIMAL BLOOD SUGAR	LOW BLOOD SUGAR
Energetic	Tired all the time
Tired when appropriate	Tired for no reason
Focused and relaxed	Restless, can't keep still
Clear	Confused
Good memory	Trouble remembering things
Able to concentrate	Trouble concentrating
Able to problem-solve effectively	Easily frustrated
Easygoing	More irritable than usual
Even-tempered	Gets angry unexpectedly

BRAIN CHEMICALS: SEROTONIN

In addition to blood sugar, there are a number of chemicals in your brain that affect how you feel and how you act. Serotonin is a brain chemical that is particularly important for sugar-sensitive people. An optimal level of serotonin creates a sense of relaxation. It mellows you out and makes you feel at peace with the world. Serotonin also influences your self-control, your impulse control, and your ability to plan ahead.

When your serotonin level is low, you may feel depressed, act impulsively, and have intense cravings for alcohol, sweets, or carbohydrates (all of which are sugars). Scientists have worked hard to find ways to increase the level of serotonin in the brains of people who are depressed. The result is that the antidepressant drugs that do this—such as Prozac, Zoloft, Paxil, Effexor, Celexa, Lexapro, and Luvox—have grown to a fourteen-*billion*-dollar industry.

Because of your inherited sugar sensitivity, you may find the symptoms of low serotonin familiar. Take a look at the next chart.

OPTIMAL LEVEL OF SEROTONIN	LOW LEVEL OF SEROTONIN
Hopeful, optimistic	Depressed
Reflective and thoughtful	Impulsive
Able to concentrate	Short attention span
Creative, focused	Blocked, scattered
Able to think things through	Flies off the handle
Able to seek help	Suicidal
Responsive	Reactive
Looks forward to dessert without an emotional charge	Craves sweets
Hungry for a variety of different foods	Craves mostly carbohydrates like bread, pasta, and cereal

BRAIN CHEMICALS: BETA-ENDORPHIN

Beta-endorphin has gotten very little attention in the books on diet, depression, or addiction. That's very strange, because it is immensely powerful. It can either drive you inexorably toward deeper addiction or raise your spirits to a level of health that you may never have known before.

When your beta-endorphin is low, you feel depressed, impulsive, and victimized. You may be touchy and tearful. Your self-esteem is low. And, perhaps worst of all, you have a desperate craving for sugar. The scientific community has been investigating beta-endorphin for more than thirty years. But the public's understanding of its effects has remained fairly limited. You may have heard of the "runner's high," a phrase that describes how the body responds to the pain of long-distance running by flooding the body with beta-endorphin, which produces a sense of euphoria.

Understanding the powerful emotional effects of beta-endorphin levels in your brain is crucial for people with sugar sensitivity. Understanding the beta-endorphin story will radically change your sense of why you feel the way you do. As you will see from the next chart, some of the effects of beta-endorphin are similar to those of serotonin.

OPTIMAL LEVEL OF BETA-ENDORPHIN	LOW LEVEL OF BETA-ENDORPHIN
High tolerance for pain	Low pain tolerance
Sensitive, sympathetic	Tearful, reactive
High self-esteem	Low self-esteem
Compassionate	Overwhelmed by others' pain
Connected and in touch	Feels isolated
Hopeful, optimistic, euphoric	Depressed, hopeless
Takes personal responsibility	Feels "done to" by others
Take-it-or-leave-it attitude toward sweet foods	Craves sugar!
Solution-oriented	Emotionally overwhelmed

As you read over the symptoms on these three charts, you may have had two reactions. You may have been comforted by recognizing patterns that sound so familiar and fit your experience so well. You may also have been amazed that your emotions and behavior can be so strongly affected by your body's chemistry.

A DELICATE BALANCE

Blood sugar, serotonin, and beta-endorphin. A normal body keeps all three in balance at optimal levels easily; a sugar-sensitive body has a harder time. Your sugar-sensitive body is likely off balance. The levels in all three of these systems must be optimal for you to conquer the Dr. Jekyll/Mr. Hyde syndrome. If you work on only one factor, the others will remain unbalanced. You will make some progress, but you will still experience the negative symptoms of having low levels of the other two factors.

Let's look at this visually. Here you are *before* making any change.

LOW BLOOD SUGAR	LOW LEVEL OF SEROTONIN	LOW LEVEL OF BETA-ENDORPHIN
Tired all the time	Depressed	Low pain tolerance
Tired for no reason	Impulsive	Tearful, reactive
Restless, can't keep still	Short attention span	Low self-esteem
Confused	Blocked, scattered	Overwhelmed by others' pain
Has trouble remembering	Flies off the handle	Feels isolated

LOW BLOOD SUGAR	LOW LEVEL OF SEROTONIN	LOW LEVEL OF BETA-ENDORPHIN
Has trouble concentrating	Suicidal	Depressed, hopeless
Easily frustrated	Reactive	Feels "done to" by others
More irritable than usual	Craves sweets	Craves sugar!
Gets angry unexpectedly	Craves mostly carbohydrates like bread, pasta, and cereal	Emotionally overwhelmed

As you can see, you feel pretty bad with all these levels out of whack. Now let's say your doctor puts you on Prozac to raise your serotonin level and ease your depression. Once you get stabilized on Prozac, you start feeling better—less depressed, more optimistic, and more focused. But you are still eating the way you always have—lots of sweets and starches. Let's see how things look now.

LOW BLOOD SUGAR	OPTIMAL LEVEL OF SEROTONIN	LOW LEVEL OF BETA-ENDORPHIN
Tired all the time	Hopeful, optimistic	Low pain tolerance
Tired for no reason	Reflective and thoughtful	Tearful, reactive
Restless, can't keep still	Able to concentrate	Low self-esteem
Confused	Creative, focused	Overwhelmed by others' pain

LOW BLOOD SUGAR	OPTIMAL LEVEL OF SEROTONIN	LOW LEVEL OF BETA-ENDORPHIN
Has trouble remembering	Able to think things through	Feels isolated
Has trouble concentrating	Able to seek help	Depressed, hopeless
Easily frustrated	Responsive	Feels "done to" by others
More irritable than usual	Looks forward to dessert a bit	Craves sugar!
Gets angry unexpectedly	Hungry for healthy foods	Emotionally overwhelmed

So although your depression is lifting, your self-esteem is still low and you feel isolated and emotionally overwhelmed. You feel better, but inside you feel that something is still missing. Something is still not right. How can you explain this? It doesn't make any sense. The Prozac is supposed to help—and it does. But why do the black feelings still come? They aren't as bad as in the past, but something is still off. And you are still exhausted at five in the afternoon.

Here is what is happening. You have raised your serotonin level, but your blood sugar and beta-endorphin levels remain low. You still get tired and feel crabby, and your self-esteem wobbles a lot. You feel isolated and overwhelmed and find it hard to concentrate. Your first thought may be that your medication isn't working. You may shift to another drug like Paxil or Zoloft, and for a while things improve. Then the same old problems come back (I'll explain why in chapter 5). But you are determined to feel better, so you keep searching for solutions.

Perhaps you come across one of the popular diet books. These books talk about needing to stabilize your blood sugar by eating more protein or by "balancing" each of your meals with a specific ratio of protein, fat, and carbohydrate. These dietary plans identify many of the symptoms you feel. So you decide to drop the medication altogether and start one of these diets. It stabilizes your blood sugar and you begin to feel better.

Here's what that looks like.

OPTIMAL BLOOD SUGAR	LOW LEVEL OF SEROTONIN	LOW LEVEL OF BETA-ENDORPHIN
Energetic	Depressed	Low pain tolerance
Tired when appropriate	Impulsive	Tearful, reactive
Focused and relaxed	Short attention span	Low self-esteem
Clear	Blocked, scattered	Overwhelmed by others' pain
Has good memory	Flies off the handle	Feels isolated
Able to concentrate	Suicidal	Depressed, hopeless
Able to solve problems effectively	Reactive	Feels "done to" by others
Easygoing	Craves sweets	Craves sugar!
Even-tempered	Craves mostly carbohydrates like bread, pasta, and cereal	Emotionally overwhelmed

Once again, you start to feel better. But trouble is coming. As it turns out, the very foods you eat that stabilize your blood sugar level will decrease your serotonin and make your low-serotonin symptoms worse. It's a terrible paradox with a terrible effect on your mood. If your diet calls for low carbs, your serotonin level will plunge. If you use sweets to create carbohydrate balance, you will make your low-beta-endorphin symptoms even worse.

One problem is that many of these new diets advocate the use of "specially balanced" nutrition bars. These bars are advertised as low-fat, natural, and healthy. But they often contain high levels of what their labels call carbohydrates. These are actually sugars that will activate your low-beta-endorphin symptoms. Chapter 5 will tell you all about how this works. These nutrition bars are very compelling for sugar-sensitive people. You may find yourself wanting to eat several bars a day. But thanks to your inherited sugar sensitivity, what starts off as convenience becomes dependence, and before you know it, you are addicted to the nutrition bars (thanks to all the sugars they contain).

However, you are on the right track in wanting to stabilize your blood sugar. If you forgo the use of nutrition bars made with sugars, stop using sugars and white-flour products (which your body reacts to like sugar), and eat complex carbohydrates (like beans or whole grains) to achieve the diet's balancing process, you can avoid the problem with your beta-endorphin.

Now things are getting better. You have improved two of the factors creating your Dr. Jekyll/Mr. Hyde syndrome. Here's where you are now (take a look at the next chart).

As you can see, this is a huge improvement. You have balanced your blood sugar and your beta-endorphin. However, you still have a problem. Within a few weeks, you will begin to feel desperate. Your depression will return with a vengeance and you will feel completely discouraged because you are doing all the right things and you still feel bad.

OPTIMAL BLOOD SUGAR	LOW LEVEL OF SEROTONIN	OPTIMAL LEVEL OF BETA-ENDORPHIN
Energetic	Depressed	High tolerance for pain
Tired when appropriate	Impulsive	Sensitive, sympathetic
Focused and relaxed	Short attention span	High self-esteem
Clear	Blocked, scattered	Compassionate
Has good memory	Flies off the handle	Connected and in touch
Able to concentrate	Suicidal	Hopeful, optimistic, euphoric
Able to solve problems effectively	Reactive	Responsive
Easygoing	Craves sweets	Take-it-or-leave-it attitude toward sweet foods
Even-tempered	Craves mostly carbohydrates like bread, pasta, and cereal	Solution-oriented

As you look at these charts, you will see how confusing it can be to make sense of what can be contradictory emotional states. If your doctor is treating you for a serotonin-type depression, but your blood sugar and beta-endorphin are imbalanced, you can still feel terrible. So your mood improves but you still feel dark. And when you try to explain this to anyone, it just sounds strange, so you stop trying. What you need is a way to address the whole problem without making yourself crazy.

Balancing the levels of all three of these important biochemicals is crucial to your well-being as a sugar-sensitive person. And you can do it with simple food and lifestyle changes. This is why my program is so mind-boggling. You do your food plan, and your body and brain do the balancing. You don't have to figure out beta-endorphin or serotonin. You just figure out breakfast.

I am fully aware that this is a profoundly outrageous concept. Especially after seeing thousands of people in my clinic get clean and sober, I believed in it enough to go back to school at age forty-eight to find out more about why. Now, ten years later, I know its truth in every cell of my being. The testimony of the hundreds of thousands of people who have done the program, in all its simplicity, and who have experienced healing have confirmed the first words written in the first edition of this book: *Your distress is caused by sugar sensitivity. I have a solution that will heal you.*

On the chart that follows you'll see the profile that can be yours by using the nutritional approach I have developed for people with inherited sugar sensitivity.

OPTIMAL BLOOD SUGAR	OPTIMAL LEVEL OF SEROTONIN	OPTIMAL LEVEL OF BETA-ENDORPHIN
Energetic	Hopeful, optimistic	High tolerance for pain
Tired when appropriate	Reflective and thoughtful	Sensitive, sympathetic
Focused and relaxed	Able to concentrate	High self-esteem
Clear	Creative, focused	Compassionate

OPTIMAL BLOOD SUGAR	OPTIMAL LEVEL OF SEROTONIN	OPTIMAL LEVEL OF BETA-ENDORPHIN
Has good memory	Able to think things through	Connected and in touch
Able to concentrate	Able to seek help	Hopeful, optimistic, euphoric
Able to solve problems effectively	Responsive	Takes personal responsibility
Easygoing	Looks forward to dessert a bit	Take-it-or-leave-it attitude toward sweet foods
Even-tempered	Hungry for healthy foods	Solution-oriented

You don't have to settle for one or two out of three. You can have optimal levels in all these vital systems. The healing process I have developed will allow you to design your own food plan, one that will specifically target your needs and personal priorities. Using it, you will learn to read your own body to see which factor is causing your symptoms. You will learn which foods contribute to your overall health and when it is best for you to eat them. As you will discover in chapter 8, when you eat is almost as important as what you eat.

Learning this process won't happen overnight. There is no magic pill that makes everything work all at once. You will have to put effort into it. But the process is very simple and you will start feeling better rapidly. As you come to understand how your blood sugar level, your serotonin level, and your beta-endorphin level affect you, you will become more and more excited about the mastery you can achieve. The Dr. Jekyll/Mr. Hyde syndrome is not a life sentence!

4

THE UPS AND DOWNS OF
BLOOD SUGAR

Because you are sugar sensitive, you respond differently to sugar than other people do. This is most immediately apparent in the effect of what you eat on your blood sugar level. While people with normal body chemistries can eat sweet foods without experiencing dramatic changes in their blood sugar level, for you the story is different. In fact, when you eat something sweet, the immediate result is not the pleasant spurt of energy caused by a *slight increase* in your blood sugar level, but all the devastating feelings brought on by a *sharp decrease* in blood sugar. Let's take a closer look.

HOW NORMAL BLOOD SUGAR WORKS

The level of sugar in your blood fluctuates with eating, sleeping, and other activities. When you eat, your blood sugar level goes up. When you use energy, your blood sugar level goes down. The most important thing for you to understand about *your* blood sugar level is that because you are sugar sensitive, it has a very powerful effect on how you feel. If your muscles or your brain can't get the blood sugar they need to perform, they will tell you very clearly that something is wrong. You may get tired, shaky, or irritable. You may have a hard time concentrating. You may forget things. You may reach for something sweet to provide a quick pick-me-up.

Most of the sugar in your blood comes from the foods you eat. The rest comes from the extra sugar stored in your liver, which is available if you run out of food for energy. The most efficient dietary source of sugar for the average person comes in the form of carbohydrates because carbs require the least amount of work by the body to convert from food to sugar in your bloodstream. Carbohydrates can either be "simple," like beer, sugar, and white flour, or they can be "complex," like potatoes, oatmeal, and whole grains. The simpler a carbohydrate is, the more quickly it can be broken down into glucose (the simplest sugar) and released into your bloodstream, where it can be carried to your cells and burned for energy. The more complex a carbohydrate is, the longer it takes to be broken down and released into the blood.

Your body's goal is to maintain the perfect level of sugar in your blood—neither too high nor too low. It uses a number of mechanisms to achieve this. First, it draws from the sugar in your blood. Your body does this by releasing a hormone called insulin, which instructs your cells to open up, draw the sugar out of your bloodstream, and pull it into themselves where it can be burned for fuel. When the level of sugar in your blood goes up, your body releases more insulin and thereby pulls more sugar into your cells. This not only provides fuel for your cells, it keeps your blood sugar level on an even keel.

If the level of sugar in your blood drops, your body will turn to the backup sugar supply stored in your liver. Your liver stores about 400 calories' worth of sugar at any given time. After this backup supply is used up, you are in trouble. Your body needs more sugar to keep functioning. It tells you to eat. Now!

For most people, this system works well. They are not even aware of the changes in their blood sugar level. However, some people are biochemically sugar sensitive. When they eat sugar, their bodies overreact by releasing far more insulin than is needed. The result is that their cells open up and pull in more sugar than they should. This causes the level of sugar in the blood to drop too low and triggers those "crazy" Mr. Hyde symptoms of low blood sugar, including fatigue, restlessness, confusion, frustration, poor memory, and irritability.

THE IMPACT OF SUGAR SENSITIVITY

Sugar-sensitive people have a more volatile blood sugar reaction to eating sweet foods than do other people. If you are sugar sensitive, your blood sugar rises more quickly and goes higher than that of other people, causing your body to release more insulin than is actually needed for the amount of food you have eaten. As a result of this spike in insulin, you experience a quicker and steeper drop in your blood sugar levels. You are more vulnerable to low blood sugar levels, also known as hypoglycemia.

Let's look at the blood sugar response of a person who is not sugar sensitive. Mary is a "normal," active working woman. She gets up, eats a breakfast of oatmeal, whole-grain toast, juice, and a cup of coffee with sweetener around 7:00 in the morning. She has a turkey sandwich, chips, and a glass of milk for lunch at around 1:00 in the afternoon, drinks a cup of tea when she gets home from work, then eats a piece of chicken, a baked potato, and green beans for dinner at about 6:30 in the evening. She has a piece of apple pie for dessert.

This is what Mary's blood sugar curve might look like:

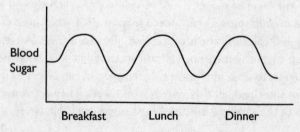

Mary's blood sugar is low when she gets up because she hasn't eaten since the night before. Her sugar level rises after breakfast and then begins to fall as her body uses the sugar for energy. The drop in her blood sugar around noon signals her body that it's time to eat. Mary recognizes these signals and has lunch. Her sugar level rises as her body digests the food she has eaten. As the sugar in that food is used for energy, her blood sugar level will begin to drop in the afternoon. When Mary eats dinner, her blood sugar rises again. After dinner and while she sleeps, her sugar level eventually drops back to where it started at the beginning of the day. Overall, her blood sugar level is pretty stable and predictable. There are no extreme peaks or valleys.

Let's look at what your blood sugar curve—as a sugar-sensitive person—might be. Your typical day might start like this. You get up at 7:00 and grab a cup of coffee with two teaspoons of sugar and some cream before you race out the door. You stop on the way to work and pick up a second cup of coffee (again with cream and sugar) and a chocolate muffin. At ten, you have another cup of coffee with two teaspoons of sugar and more cream. You are so busy working that you forget to eat lunch. At 3:00 in the afternoon, you get really tired and feel as if you are going to "fall off the cliff," so you go to the deli downstairs and get a pasta salad and some iced tea. At 4:30 you are really sleepy so you get a Coke from the machine. You get home at 7:00, pour yourself a glass of wine to unwind, and watch the news. You poke around the refrigerator for something to eat. Finding nothing, you boil water, cook some pasta, put butter and cheese on it, and eat it while watching TV. At 9:00 you get the munchies so you fetch a bag of cookies and a glass of milk.

Let's take your day a piece at a time and I'll explain what's going on behind the scenes. This graph shows your blood sugar rising after having the coffee and muffin (see graph next page).

As you now know, sugar-sensitive people overreact to eating simple carbohydrates; your blood sugar goes up higher and goes up more quickly than other people's. The sugar in your coffee and the chocolate muffin create a blood sugar spike and your body gets the

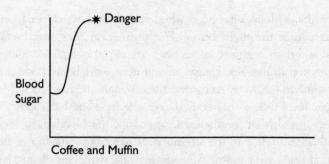

message that something is wrong. It registers DANGER! and goes into action to get the extra sugar out of your blood. Your body wants to maintain the correct level of sugar within your blood. If there is too much, your pancreas will release insulin to move the sugar from your blood into your cells. If your blood sugar spike is big, your body will tell your pancreas to release a big hit of insulin, which instructs your cells to open up and grab the sugar. You experience a rapid and steep drop in your blood sugar level.

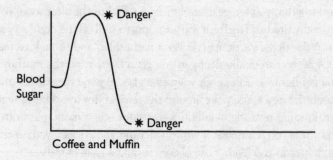

Because of this big hit of insulin, your blood sugar drops dramatically, and your body *again* registers DANGER! and gets mobilized to find a solution. This time the danger comes from having too little sugar in your blood. Whether consciously or unconsciously, you start looking for something to raise your blood sugar level quickly. Desperate to find something sweet, you drink more coffee with sugar in it. You can guess what happens now with your blood sugar level. It shoots up again. And the insulin process begins again.

If you chart these ups and downs during the day, they might look like this:

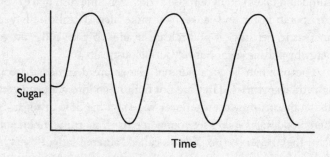

You can see that your body experiences these dramatic peaks and valleys several times a day. What are the consequences of these wild fluctuations in your blood sugar level? The first is simple. Your moods, like your blood sugar, fluctuate all day. Sometimes you feel high and sometimes you feel low. You may feel focused and alert for thirty minutes after eating, but then you can't remember who you are talking to on the phone. Or your problem-solving skills suddenly desert you and you haven't a clue how to cope with the emergency that just came up. Your Dr. Jekyll/Mr. Hyde symptoms change with the change in your blood sugar levels. (Sometimes I wonder if the vial that Dr. Jekyll drank was filled with sugar.) What do you think your own blood sugar curve would look like if you plotted it throughout the day?

ADRENAL FATIGUE

In addition to these Dr. Jekyll/Mr. Hyde mood swings, there is another repercussion from having your blood sugar rise and fall dramatically. Each time your blood sugar spikes so quickly, your body's internal alarms start ringing and signal your adrenal glands to release adrenaline, the hormone that gives us a quick surge of energy and mobilizes us in the face of danger. This response kept our ancestors alive when they were being chased by saber-toothed tigers. You can feel that zing today when you have a near-miss accident while driving to work or when someone comes up from behind and takes you by surprise. The adrenaline rush makes your heart pump faster and makes you more alert. (It also tells your pancreas to get in gear and release insulin so your cells can get energy by pulling sugar out of your bloodstream.)

The problem is, your adrenal glands are designed for coping with *emergencies*. They are not built to go into action several times a day, as they do whenever you eat a big dose of sugar. So when blood sugar spikes set your adrenals off morning, noon, and night, they begin to tire. What's called "adrenal fatigue" sets in. When that happens, your adrenals respond more slowly to the danger signal. Instead of catching the rapidly rising blood sugar early, they go into action late.

Think of the adrenals as a volunteer firefighter who has been working overtime for three months. He is totally exhausted. The alarm bell rings at 3:00 in the morning. Instead of leaping out of bed, he vaguely hears the alarm, struggles to focus, finally recognizes that it is the fire bell ringing rather than his dream, stumbles out of bed, gropes for his boots, walks to his truck, slumps at the wheel, then finally gets mobilized to turn the motor on and get to the fire. He used to leap from his bed, drop his feet into his boots in an instant, and be out the door before the bell had finished ringing. But his fatigue is clobbering his response time.

Because your adrenals are reacting late, your blood sugar rises even higher and your body releases even more insulin in an attempt to get that sugar out of your blood and into your cells. The result is that the peaks and valleys in your blood sugar level get steeper and the interval between them gets shorter. Your blood sugar curve starts to look like this:

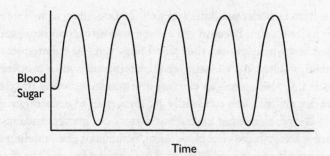

Ironically, adrenal fatigue—which is caused by your body's over-reaction to sugar—means you need more sugar more often because you drop into the lower danger zone more and more frequently. Thus adrenal fatigue makes your blood sugar ups and downs even *more* pronounced and some of your Dr. Jekyll/Mr. Hyde symptoms may get even worse. You may not be aware that this change for the worse is related to what you eat and when you eat it. You may think your bad feelings are caused by stress, lack of sleep, or PMS. Think about how often you experience the following symptoms:

☑ Fatigue

☑ Restlessness

☑ Confusion

☑ Shakiness

☑ Frustration

☑ Irritability

☑ Difficulty remembering

☑ Anger (men)

☑ Feeling weepy (women)

☑ Feeling anxious

It's no wonder you don't feel well. You are riding a physiological roller coaster. Because you are sugar sensitive and because of what and when you eat, your blood sugar can't be counted on to remain stable and give you a reliable and steady source of energy. By 3:00 in the afternoon, you feel as if you are crawling through the day. By 7:00, you can hardly get it together to make dinner.

The problem is not in your mind. It is not a matter of attitude. Unless you stabilize your blood sugar, no amount of counseling or insight will help you feel better. That's the bad news. The good news is that you can solve this problem by understanding three things:

1. Which foods will give you a stable blood sugar level that will not send your adrenal glands into action unnecessarily
2. Which foods will evoke the least reactive insulin response
3. When to eat to keep your energy up and your spirits high

In the next chapter we'll look at the two other key players in defeating your body's sugar sensitivity, the brain chemicals serotonin and beta-endorphin. Then you'll start putting into action a food plan that can give you the emotional stability and high self-esteem you've wanted—and deserved—for so long.

5

BRAIN CHEMISTRY 101

While eliminating extreme highs and lows in your blood sugar level can have a hugely positive effect on how you feel, getting your blood sugar stable will not solve all the problems of the Dr. Jekyll/Mr. Hyde syndrome. If it could, you would not need to read this book. A number of experts have written on the importance of optimal blood sugar levels for emotional well-being, but there's more to our sugar sensitivity story, and it includes some vital information that has not been widely available to the public before. This information is about the crucial importance of beta-endorphin, one of the brain chemicals we discussed briefly in chapter 3.

Serotonin and beta-endorphin can have dramatically positive—or negative—effects on your moods and your energy level. These brain chemicals work in a way that is a little more complex than the mechanics of blood sugar, and you will need some background about how the brain works to understand it. If you'd rather skip the details about the science and get started on your food plan, turn to chapter 6. As you design your plan, I will show you which of the seven steps for implementing the plan will affect your serotonin and beta-endorphin levels, as well as your blood sugar level. That way, you can return to the material in this chapter as you reach each step.

In the long run, however, taking the time now to learn about how your brain works will provide you with a real sense of confidence. It will help you to understand the nuances of what you are feeling and the reasons why you are feeling them. You can learn the difference between feelings based on serotonin versus feelings based on beta-endorphin. This ability to identify the specific physiological changes driving your feelings and behavior becomes incredibly exciting. It puts you in the driver's seat and gives you a way to direct your life as you never have before. When you add to this learning process through a dialogue with others who are doing the program, it is even more powerful. As I have seen time and again with my clients, having an exhilarating feeling of self-confidence is well worth the effort to understand the science.

We'll begin the chapter by taking a look at neurotransmitters, the family of brain chemicals to which serotonin and beta-endorphin belong. I'll explain the purpose of neurotransmitters, the mechanism by which they send information between brain cells, and the adjustments the brain makes to keep this information flow a steady one. Then we'll look at each of these neurotransmitters separately and examine how traditional drugs, both prescription and nonprescription, affect them. Finally, I will discuss why and how using food can provide an ideal way for balancing your brain chemistry.

NEUROTRANSMITTERS: MESSENGERS OF THE BRAIN

Your brain is designed to communicate information. Billions of brain cells talk to each other moment by moment through a complex network of interconnecting cells. These cells do not actually touch one another. There is a tiny space between each of them, and information is passed across this space by way of chemical *messengers* called neurotransmitters. The brain chemicals serotonin and beta-endorphin, which, as we saw in chapter 3, have such a powerful effect on your moods and behavior, are two types of neurotransmitters.

There are many kinds of neurotransmitters, each of which has a different molecular shape and carries its own distinct message. When one brain cell wants to send a message to another, it releases the appropriate type of chemical messenger into the space between it and the receiving cell. These neurotransmitters float across this tiny channel and look for a place to land.

Each receiving cell has thousands of receptors ready to catch neurotransmitters. These cells are called neuroreceptors, and each is designed to match a specific neurotransmitter. A molecule of serotonin, for example, can pass its message only to a serotonin *receptor*. The same is true with beta-endorphin. If any other kind of neurotransmitter hits the beta-endorphin receptors, nothing happens. But when the neurotransmitter that fits the receptor comes along, the receptor recognizes it and allows the message to pass. If enough receptors get the same message, then the entire cell responds and passes the message to the next cell. Of course, this all happens in a very, very short time. Let's look at how this communication works with our two neurotransmitters.

First, here's an example of how beta-endorphin, which eases physical and emotional pain, works. Susan drops a heavy box on her fingers. Her first response is one of intense pain. She is nauseous and feels like she will pass out. However, before too long, this passes and she feels clear and focused. Her fingers still hurt, but she knows what to do. She knows that ice will reduce the swelling and help to numb the pain.

While Susan is standing at the sink with her fingers in a bowl of ice water, she is surprised to notice that she feels a little relaxed and spacey. This seems strange since she just smashed her fingers. But Susan's brain recognized a crisis when the pain sensations started to reach it and responded by releasing beta-endorphin molecules that blunted those throbbing sensations.

Let's take an even closer look at this painkilling mechanism. Susan's beta-endorphin molecules are stored in her brain cells.

When the sending cells recognized "pain," they released beta-endorphin. The beta-endorphin molecules crossed the space between brain cells and hit the beta-endorphin receptors on the receiving cells, causing the cell to receive the message and respond to it. Because Susan felt a lot of pain, a lot of beta-endorphin was released and a powerful "Block that pain!" message got through.

While the neurotransmitter beta-endorphin deals with pain, serotonin deals with mood and behavior. Let's look at another example. Diane is sugar sensitive. She is also a compulsive eater and she loves certain foods. She often talks about wanting to lose weight, but when she goes out to a restaurant one evening and bread appears on the table while she is waiting for her dinner to be served, her resolve evaporates. Diane has low levels of serotonin, the neurotransmitter that puts the brakes on impulses. Because she is sugar sensitive, Diane's behavior "brakes" don't always work.

If Diane had the body chemistry of a normal person, her brain would have an adequate level of serotonin, which would enable her to recognize the message to "eat bread now" as impulsive behavior (as opposed to actual hunger) and not act on it. But because Diane's serotonin levels are naturally low, there is less of it flowing between her brain cells. The small amount of serotonin she has crosses the space between her brain cells, finds the serotonin receptors, and passes along the message to "stop," which should defuse Diane's impulse to eat. But because there isn't very much serotonin, the message remains pretty weak. Not enough of the receptors are activated, so the cells don't pass the message along, and Diane's impulse to eat the bread is not quieted. Instead she practically inhales the bread, eating way more than she really wants to.

Let's imagine that we have now increased Diane's serotonin levels. She still feels bad about her eating patterns and still looks at the bread on her table, saying to herself, "I will just have a little of this bread while I am waiting." But before she pops a piece into her mouth, something happens. A little voice says, "Wait a minute, Diane. Are you sure that's the best thing to do?" So Diane thinks about it a little. She sighs and thinks, "Well, um, maybe that's not such a good idea." Diane has just exercised impulse control, courtesy of serotonin.

When we increased Diane's imaginary serotonin level, there were many more serotonin molecules hitting the serotonin receptors, and the cells passed the message throughout her brain, in effect telling Diane to "wait." Diane's impulse quieted down as the message got through. Diane got another benefit from increasing her level of serotonin: her feelings of irritability, isolation, and depression were quieted as well. Diane didn't understand how all this worked in her brain. She didn't have a clue about the serotonin action. And she didn't need to. She just felt more in control of her life and her behavior. Diane's brain knew exactly what it was doing, though: more serotonin equals impulse control and better feelings.

Later, you'll learn how to safely increase your serotonin and beta-endorphin levels by changing the foods you eat and doing other things like exercise, meditation or prayer, laughter, and even having good sex!

CLEANING UP AND REGULATING THE SYSTEM

After a neurotransmitter lands in its own receptor and passes its message along, it floats back into the space between brain cells and is available to hit the receptor again. At the same time, the sending cell keeps releasing more of the same neurotransmitter. This creates a risk of overload. To prevent this, your brain has a couple of ways to get rid of the "leftover" serotonin and beta-endorphin molecules.

First, it releases enzymes that break down the used neurotransmitters. I like to think of each enzyme as a little Pacman chomping the used neurotransmitters. The other mechanism that prevents neurotransmitter overload is a sort of vacuum cleaner that sucks up the used messengers and deposits them back in the sending cell to be recycled for later use. These "vacuum cleaners" are called reuptake pumps. Like the Pacman enzymes, the reuptake pumps are usually very effective. Your brain not only wants things cleaned up, it also wants them orderly and organized. That's why the brain's system of neurotransmitters and neuroreceptors is carefully orchestrated to stay in balance. If things get unbalanced, your brain will try to compensate for the problem. Three of these adjustments are particularly important to our story. These are downregulation, upregulation, and withdrawal.

Downregulation

Receiving too much of any given message confuses your brain. It doesn't like being overloaded. For example, if too much of a given neurotransmitter is released, the receiving cell will close down some of its receptors, thereby limiting the number of hits it can receive. Even though there are more neurotransmitters released, there are fewer places for them to land. This process of closing down receptors is called downregulation.

Downregulation is what causes people to develop a tolerance to a drug. Let's use painkilling drugs as an example. Painkillers like morphine work because their molecules are shaped like beta-endorphin molecules and they fit into the beta-endorphin receptors. This is how they pass along the painkilling message. But when you take a painkilling drug, you get many more painkilling "hits" than you would normally. So your brain, which values balance above all else, wants to get things back to "normal." After a while it will close down some of its receptors. In other words, it downregulates. Downregulation results in your brain cells getting fewer hits. This is why the same amount of your painkiller has less and less effect over time. This is how you develop a "tolerance" for a drug and need a bigger dose to get the same effect. Downregulation happens fairly quickly. You might need 50 mg of morphine to get relief from pain on the first day and 500 mg of morphine to achieve the same effect ten days later.

Just as painkillers work on the beta-endorphin system, anti-depressants work on the serotonin system. When Barbara started taking Prozac for depression, she was prescribed 20 mg a day. After getting over some initial side effects, she felt a whole lot better for a few months. The Prozac was increasing the number of serotonin "hits" in her brain. Then her depression returned. Her doctor upped the dosage to 40 mg a day and Barbara felt better again. But over time, the bad feelings started creeping back in. This was because Barbara's brain had downregulated in response to the increase in the serotonin "hits" caused by the Prozac so it now had less of an effect. Here's a picture to show you how down-regulation works.

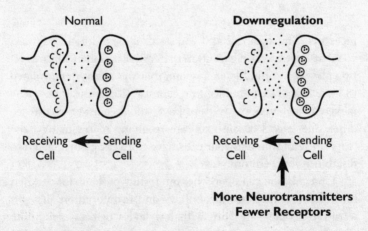

Upregulation

The brain chemistry balancing system works in the other direction as well. If your level of serotonin or beta-endorphin gets too low, your brain will open up more receptors so it can get more hits. The picture on page 70 shows upregulation.

Upregulation creates some interesting problems. If you are sugar sensitive and have naturally low levels of serotonin, then your system has already upregulated to have more serotonin

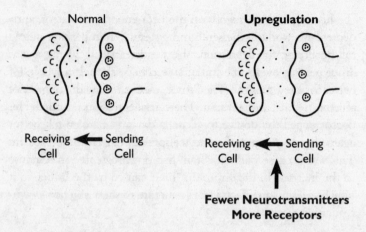

Normal

Upregulation

Receiving ◄── Sending
Cell   Cell

Receiving ◄── Sending
Cell   Cell

**Fewer Neurotransmitters
More Receptors**

receptors. This means that if you start taking a drug like Prozac, you may have a very big reaction to it. All of a sudden you are getting more serotonin hits in a system that was already upregulated to have lots of extra serotonin receptors. Taking the Prozac may make you feel anxious or jittery, have wild dreams, or experience other side effects because you are receiving many, many more "hits" of serotonin and your cells have not yet downregulated to restabilize your serotonin level.

Upregulation causes another interesting problem for children of alcoholics. Children of alcoholics—and, in my opinion, all sugar-sensitive people—are born with low levels of beta-endorphin, so their brains are normally in an upregulated state to compensate: they have more beta-endorphin receptors than normal. This means they can overreact to any substance that evokes a beta-endorphin response. Let's take a look at an example from one of my clients.

Joe is a twelve-year-old child of an alcoholic and has low levels of beta-endorphin. On the outside he acts "cool" when hanging out with his buddies, but inside he doesn't feel too good about himself. One day, Joe and his buddies sneak a six-pack of beer. His buddies have normal brain chemistry. They drink a can of beer or two and feel good, slightly high and pretty relaxed.

But Joe's brain has far more beta-endorphin receptors because his own natural level of beta-endorphin is low. So when Joe drinks two cans of beer, POW! The alcohol causes a release of beta-endorphin with its capacity for easing emotional pain. Joe is on top of the world. He feels better than he has in his whole life because his extra receptors have amplified the effect of the beta-endorphin release caused by the alcohol in the beer. "This is great!" Joe says. And will he drink again? You bet he will. He will probably spend the rest of his life seeking to relive the euphoria of his first drink.

Withdrawal

The third way your brain tries to recover from imbalance is by creating withdrawal symptoms. When you develop a physical dependence on a substance—such as a morphine-based pain-killer, alcohol, or sugar—you have altered the natural state of your system. Your brain gets used to having the extra serotonin or beta-endorphin hits caused by the substance and it "complains" if the substance is cut off. You experience these complaints as withdrawal symptoms such as irritability, headaches, diarrhea, joint pain, and other flulike symptoms.

When you are experiencing withdrawal and you take the substance your neuroreceptors are screaming for, you immediately feel better—at least for a little while. This rapid improvement is one of the best ways to test whether the feelings you are experiencing come from physical (as opposed to emotional) dependency and withdrawal. If you immediately feel better when you give your body what it craves, it's a strong clue that you are dealing with physical dependency and withdrawal.

Now that you have a better sense of the overall chemistry affecting your brain process, let's take a deeper look at the specific neurotransmitters affecting the sugar-sensitive person.

SEROTONIN

As we saw in chapter 3, when your serotonin level is in an ideal state, you feel mellow and relaxed. You feel at peace with life. Serotonin also increases your impulse control, which allows you to more easily "just say no." People with low levels of serotonin do not have good impulse control. It is almost impossible for them to "just say no" because there is such a short time period between the urge to do something and doing it. This is why the warm cookies on the kitchen table hop into your mouth before you even know what has happened. This is why no matter how many times you vow to stick with your diet, you are not able to. The insufficient serotonin level in your brain isn't giving you the time you need to make good decisions.

Besides being impulsive, people with low levels of serotonin can feel depressed and crave simple carbohydrates such as bread, pasta, or candy. When your brain is low in serotonin, it works to do whatever it can to increase it. Not only does it upregulate, or open up more receptors to grab whatever serotonin your brain cells are releasing, it also produces cravings for foods that will raise your serotonin level, which simple carbohydrates can do.

Here's how. Your body makes serotonin from a chemical called tryptophan. Tryptophan is an amino acid that comes from protein. But, although eating turkey, for example, will get tryptophan into your blood, this doesn't necessarily mean it will get into your brain to be made into serotonin. You need the chemical properties of simple carbohydrates to move the tryptophan out of your bloodstream and into your brain where it can be used to make serotonin. We'll talk more about how to use tryptophan to raise your spirits, improve your sleep, and help you feel more relaxed in chapter 9, but for now remember that snacking on a carbohydrate can raise the level of serotonin in your brain only if you've eaten enough protein first to get tryptophan into your bloodstream.

This fact has encouraged a number of authors to recommend eating sweets—and in particular chocolate—as the ideal alternative to antidepressant drugs. I strongly disagree. Though chocolate does raise serotonin levels, it is not the best solution for raising your serotonin levels *and* relieving depression. Chocolate may work for someone else, but not for you. You are sugar sensitive. When you eat chocolate, you will get a rise in your serotonin level, but at a huge price. Chocolate will backfire on you by increasing your craving for sweets and reinforcing your addiction. You'll see why this happens when we get to the section on beta-endorphin.

How Antidepressants Work

Another school of thought says that the best way to raise low serotonin levels—and thereby relieve depression—is to take an antidepressant drug. Most antidepressants work by increasing the amount of serotonin received by the neuroreceptors. The scientists who developed antidepressants focused on creating drugs that would cause the original low number of serotonin molecules released by a depressed person's brain cells to remain in the space between the cells for a longer time, thus allowing these molecules to hit the serotonin receptors more than once. There are antidepressants that do this by blocking the little Pacman enzyme that gobbles up extra serotonin. Other antidepressants work by stopping the reuptake pumps from vacuuming up the used neurotransmitters.

Drugs called SSRIs (selective serotonin reuptake inhibitors), such as Prozac, Paxil, Effexor, Celexa, and Zoloft belong to the second type. They turn off the reuptake pumps so the used serotonin stays in the space between the cells and continues to hit the serotonin receptors. In effect, your brain is getting more use out of the serotonin you have. These antidepressants tend to work better than the Pacman-blocking kind because they have fewer side effects.

The good thing about drugs like Prozac is that they do increase your serotonin level and improve the problem moods and behaviors associated with low serotonin. As we saw in chapter 3, higher levels of serotonin make you less depressed, less scattered, more focused, less blocked, less irritable, and less likely to crave sweets, bread, pasta, or cereal. Thanks to the improved impulse control that serotonin gives you, you are also better able to say no to alcohol, food, and compulsive behaviors.

As with the chocolate "solution," however, there are significant problems with the antidepressant solution. First, as we saw in Barbara's case, your brain will close down some serotonin receptors after a while to return the serotonin level in your brain to its "normal" pre-antidepressant level (which, in your case is too low). Then you will have to increase your dose or change the type of medication you are using to get the same effect. Second, many of these drugs are very expensive and must be taken under the supervision of a psychiatrist, a situation that may not be covered by your health insurance. And third, even the newer antidepressants have unpleasant side effects. You may experience nausea, jitteriness, weird dreams, or problems with your sleep. You may find that you have no sex drive, are less sensitive physically to sexual stimulation, and cannot achieve orgasm. While antidepressants can be life saving if you have a serious depression that does not respond to anything else, the side effects can be a high price to pay for this relief.

There are other options. Certain ways of eating can significantly alter your serotonin levels. What and when you eat can be a wonderful ally in your process. If you eat a baked potato (with the skin) as a snack before bed, you will put the biochemistry in motion to get the tryptophan into your brain to make serotonin. As you continue to read this book, you will begin to see why potatoes may be a better alternative than Prozac.

BETA-ENDORPHIN

Let's turn to the next neurotransmitter important to sugar-sensitive people, beta-endorphin. Beta-endorphin acts as a powerful natural painkiller. I've mentioned the "runner's high" (also called an "endorphin rush"), where the body responds to the pain of long-distance running by flooding the brain with soothing beta-endorphin. Your natural beta-endorphin is incredibly potent and serves you well. The problem for sugar-sensitive people, however, is that their "normal" level of beta-endorphin may be low and their natural response to a beta-endorphin-releasing substance (like sugar) may be significantly greater than that of people with ordinary body chemistry. As we'll see later, that can cause huge problems.

In scientific terms, beta-endorphin is an "endogenous opioid," which means that it can be found naturally in the body and has an opium-like effect such as that of heroin and morphine. Like the other opioids, beta-endorphin (at the proper level) produces a sense of well-being, reduces pain, eases emotional distress, increases self-esteem, creates emotional stability, and even produces a feeling of euphoria. Not surprisingly, beta-endorphin also controls anxiety, defuses paranoid feelings, reduces anger, and relieves certain types of depression. With all these positive effects coming from sufficient beta-endorphin, you can see the problems you run into when your system isn't producing enough. If your beta-endorphin level is naturally low, you will have to live with low self-esteem that is *biochemically* based and therefore won't respond to psychotherapy, counseling, self-help books, or positive affirmations.

Narcotics such as morphine, heroin, and codeine work like beta-endorphin because their molecules have the same shape. They can fit into beta-endorphin receptors and fool the brain into thinking that more natural beta-endorphin was sent. The result is the same as that produced by natural beta-endorphin: a high tolerance for pain, a feeling of euphoria, optimism, and high self-esteem.

As we saw in the case of Joe, alcohol also has a beta-endorphin effect in the brain. It does not act on the receptors directly as narcotics do. Instead it causes the brain to release additional beta-endorphin to produce the "high" we associate with drinking. And since we sugar-sensitive people have naturally lower levels of beta-endorphins, our brains are normally upregulated.

That is, they have opened up more receptors to receive the few beta-endorphins that are usually there—so we get an even bigger high from drinking than many of our buddies. Like Joe, we tend to really like the effect that alcohol produces. Sugar-sensitive people have a bigger reaction to all the things that evoke a beta-endorphin response, as we will see.

Sugar and the Beta-endorphin Response

Let's go back to our old friend sugar in the context of this heightened beta-endorphin response. Like alcohol, sugar causes a release of beta-endorphin. It can make you feel high. It can reduce both physical and emotional pain. Normal people can enjoy this property of sugar without ill effects. But a sugar-sensitive person responds to the beta-endorphin effect of sugar in a much bigger way because their brain naturally has many more beta-endorphin receptors. For a sugar-sensitive person, eating sugar can feel like drinking alcohol! Sugar can make us funny, relaxed, silly, inappropriate, talkative, and (temporarily) self-confident.

There have been a number of scientists and physicians who have been interested in how sugar affects our minds and bodies. In fact, people have been writing about the harmful effects of sugar since the early 1950s. But most of these publications weren't taken seriously by the medical community. They tended to be dismissed as "unscientific" and "anecdotal."

In the mid-1980s, scientists started looking at sugars in a more focused way. Dr. Elliott Blass conducted some fascinating experiments that looked at the possibility of using sugar as a safe analgesic (painkiller) for babies. To test his hypothesis that sugar could be used in this way, Blass timed the reactions of a group of mice exposed to a potentially painful level of heat. He first rested the front foot of a mouse on a hot plate and then measured how quickly it lifted its paw from the heat. The mice lifted their little feet up in an average of 10 seconds. Blass then gave the mice a drink that was 11.5 percent sugar and repeated the experiment.

This time it took them an average of 20 seconds—twice as long—to lift those tiny paws. These results suggested that the sugar was blocking the pain of the heat; it was acting like a painkiller.

Blass then tried to establish the neurochemical basis for what he was seeing. He had observed that the ingestion of sugar was reducing the mice's pain response, but he wasn't sure which neurochemical pathway was involved. It was Blass's belief that the sugar somehow acted like an opioid—perhaps by causing a release of the natural painkiller beta-endorphin—so he designed an experiment using the drug Naltrexone to test his hypothesis. Naltrexone, which blocks the painkilling effect of opioid drugs such as morphine and heroin, works by sitting in the beta-endorphin receptors and preventing them from receiving the soothing, painkilling message that beta-endorphin wants to transmit to the body. Blass reasoned that if Naltrexone also blocked the painkilling effect of sugar (which he would learn by observing how quickly mice given Naltrexone reacted to the hot plate), it would mean that sugar acted on the brain—specifically, the beta-endorphin system—like an opioid.

In his new experiment, Blass gave the mice a dose of Naltrexone before giving them the sugar drink. Then he tested their reaction to the hot plate. The mice picked up their little feet real quickly. This time those little paws were up in eight seconds, as if they were saying, "That thing is HOT!!!" The Naltrexone had indeed blocked the painkilling effect of the sugar. Because Naltrexone works only on the beta-endorphin system, this experiment showed that sugar affects the brain by stimulating a beta-endorphin release, the same way opioid drugs do. This study provided evidence that sugar works like a drug to block pain.

Sugar and Isolation Distress

In 1986, the same year that Blass did the experiments on sugar and physical pain, he also reported results from an experiment on sugar and emotional pain, in which he measured the effect of sugar on what's called "isolation distress." "Isolation distress" is a scientific term that describes the emotional stress of animals when they are separated from their mothers and left alone.

Blass measured isolation distress in little mouse pups by measuring how many times they cried during the test period. When the pups were with Mama mouse, they didn't cry. When they were taken away from Mama, they started crying big time. The eight pups who were given nothing to soothe them cried more than 300 times in a six-minute period. The eight pups who were given sugar water cried only about 75 times in the same period. Next, Blass gave the pups a dose of Naltrexone before giving them sugar water and—just like in the hot plate experiment—the Naltrexone blocked the soothing effect of the sugar and the second batch of little pups cried as often as those who hadn't had the sugar. Apparently the sugar was blocking *emotional* pain just as it had blocked physical pain.

Sugar and Learned Helplessness

Since Blass's experiments, scientists have continued to look at the effects of sugar on the mind and body. Most of this work has been done in the context of alcoholism research. Since both sugar and alcohol evoke a beta-endorphin response, a number of studies have linked the preference for sweets to a preference for alcohol. Scientists have clearly shown that alcoholic mice—mice that have been bred to prefer alcohol—really go for sweets. But there's more, and it has to do with other ways beta-endorphin affects your behavior.

This part of the story starts with Dr. Christine Gianoulakis at McGill University, who noticed that two different strains of lab mice responded to alcohol in two very different ways. One group, the C57GL/6 mice, had a far more intense reaction than their brothers and sisters, the DBA/2 mice. When Dr. Gianoulakis and her colleagues looked for the reason why, they discovered that C57s are born with much lower levels of beta-endorphin in their brains. So, just like you, the C57s' brains increase the number of beta-endorphin receptor sites (in other words, they upregulate) to try to catch more of whatever beta-endorphin is available. Then, because the C57s have more places to catch the beta-endorphin, they get a bigger response to things—like alcohol—that cause a release of beta-endorphin. (What's more, the C57s not only responded to alcohol more powerfully than the DBA mice, they had a reaction to morphine that was *thirty-five times more powerful*. Think of that.)

The sugar story and its effect on C57s are well researched throughout the scientific literature. Dr. Gianoulakis later extended her study from mice to men and looked at the children and grandchildren of alcoholics, who are known to be genetically predisposed to alcohol addiction. They, too, start out with lower levels of beta-endorphin and have a heightened response to alcohol and sugars, things that evoke beta-endorphin.

In the first edition of *Potatoes Not Prozac*, I went a step further than the studies and asked, *"What if sugar-sensitive people are the human equivalent of the C57 mouse strain?"* If you follow the similarities, you will begin to see why some people seek sugar, love sugar, and get addicted to sugar. The resemblance is extraordinary. If you start thinking of yourself as a big C57 mouse, you get *lots* of clues about why you act the way you do. And you can understand why your DBA friends cannot in any way understand why you keep going back to sugars when they just say no.

Science also offers some good insight about our attitudes toward the different types of mice (or people). Scientists do not look down upon the little C57s. Nor do they laud the DBAs. They simply know that these are two very distinct strains of mice with two very different body chemistries. There's no moral judgment involved. You can do the same thing by taking the negative judgment and shame off your C57 way of life. The first step is understanding that this is a biochemical process. Now that you understand how your brain chemistry works, you can start making choices for healing.

Here are some of the findings that have been published about C57 mice. Take a look and then we'll reflect on what these studies might mean for your healing.

1. All C57s, regardless of gender, like sweet stuff more than DBAs.
2. When something bad or scary happens, DBAs look for an escape, while C57s crouch, become immobile and defensive. The C57 behavior is called "defeat-induced learned submission," and it occurs in response to a release of beta-endorphin.
3. The "defeated" mice developed a tolerance to the beta-endorphin released in response to a threat.
4. Morphine makes C57s hyperactive but *does not* have the same effect on DBAs.
5. When withdrawing from morphine, C57s become lethargic and passive.

Let's translate these into your own experience. We'll replace the word C57 with "a sugar-sensitive person." And, since we know morphine and sugar both affect your beta-endorphin receptors, let's replace the word morphine with "sugar." Now we'll go through the list again.

1. *All sugar-sensitive people, regardless of gender, like sweet stuff more than people with nonsugar-sensitive bodies.*
   You all know some people who act like DBAs. They are the ones who say to us, "Why don't you just say no?" They are the ones who decide to diet, and do, and then lose ten pounds in a month. They are the ones who give up chocolate for Lent and never look back, the ones who carried a little orange pumpkin at Halloween instead of a giant sack. They are the ones who would eat the warm chocolate chip cookie on the kitchen counter only if they were hungry. You know immediately who they are. Since society tends to recognize and value DBA behavior, you may judge yourself against their standard.

You may believe that DBA behavior is good and C57 behavior is bad.

2. *When something bad or scary happens, a sugar-sensitive person crouches, becomes immobile and defensive. This behavior is called "defeat-induced learned submission," and it occurs in response to a release of beta-endorphin.*

When you feel defeated and overwhelmed, you assume the fetal position, lie still, and tell everyone it is not your fault. Now, you may not do this on the outside. On the outside you may do big theater and have everyone believe that you are absolutely in control. But inside you are holding on by a thread and feeling horrible. When there's a crisis, you may be lying still—way inside your heart instead of visibly—but you absolutely know this pattern. In psychological terms, this is called "learned helplessness." You don't see your DBA friends respond like this to the same crises. They get mobilized and energized. You take Prozac; they change jobs and get a promotion. You hate this "injustice" and have not a clue how biochemically mediated it is.

3. *The "defeated" mice developed a tolerance to the beta-endorphin released in response to a threat.*

If you have experienced a lifetime of defeat, you become numb to it. You don't notice it anymore, and you expect defeat as part of life. You have no sense at all that this is biochemically driven. You just think you got dealt a bad hand in life and this is your lot. You turn to sweets for comfort and solace. When your DBA friends experience defeat, they simply see it as a temporary setback and not an expected life pattern. And they take action to move around it and go forward.

4. *Sugar makes sugar-sensitive people hyperactive, but does* not *have the same effect on nonsugar-sensitive people.*

Sweet foods give you "energy" and lift you out of the lethargy of beta-endorphin withdrawal. Sweet foods can also give you motor mouth. You become engaging, funny, and self-confident. Sometimes friends wonder if you have been drinking. More often than not, you've chosen other sugar-sensitive people as friends, so you go out for coffee, have cake, and really enjoy your social time. Having coffee with the sweets feels like heaven. You get clear, focused, and relaxed—for about thirty minutes. You love that feeling. And those cold, frosty, sugary coffee drinks (you know which ones I mean) are the best because they make you feel so energized. Your DBA friends enjoy their coffee (they have a plain bagel with it), but they do not live for it. You see these same behaviors in your children and grandchildren. Give a sugar-sensitive three-year-old a piece of birthday cake and he will be the life of the party. Give a sugar-sensitive two-year-old a twelve-ounce can of Sprite on the plane and she will be bouncing over the top of the seat for two hours. The more work you do with your program, the more clearly you will see this profound shift in behavior (yours and that of others) before and after eating sugar.

5. *When withdrawing from sugar, sugar-sensitive people become lethargic and passive.*
When you try to detox from sugar, you sit around and wait till it's over. You hunker down with your discomfort. You are immobile. You feel as if your cells are literally made of lead and/or you feel as if they are all screaming. You experience the effects of withdrawal in your gut, your skin, and your brain—wherever there are beta-endorphin receptor sites.

Pretty interesting, isn't it? For years you have struggled with learned helplessness, with self-esteem that fades in moments. You vacillate between hyperactive clarity and lying on the couch in a stupor. The Dr. Jeykll/Mr. Hyde syndrome hits very close to home. But I am pushing you beyond the idea of mood swings. I am inviting you to think of yourself as a big C57 mouse and connect with the enormity of what these mouse studies mean for us.

If you are sugar sensitive, you have no doubt experienced druglike effects after eating sugar. Unfortunately, this response is not usually taken seriously. People make jokes about being a "chocoholic," but they rarely speak of the real pain caused by their continuing and compulsive use of sweets. Now that you know the C57 story, you can really get that all those things you thought were character flaws are a function of your sugar-sensitive biochemistry.

> Before the program, I was always trying to set rules about how each day was run—quite rigid ones like "I am going to exercise for one hour every day." I made all kinds of plans—daily plans, weekly plans, monthly plans, plans of plans . . . And, frankly, I never managed to stick with or do any of them. I always felt like an undisciplined failure, especially when I could see that other people seemed to be able to pick something to do and just do it. Also, my plans were grandiose. It was never "I'll read a book"; it was "I'll read a book a week for the whole year." Now if I get grandiose, I know it means my program is wobbly.
>
> —Vinny

While scientists slowly continue to explore the relationship of sugar to addiction, you can draw from your own experience as a sugar-sensitive person to see how powerful a "drug" sugar can be. You know how big an impact the soothing beta-endorphin release triggered by sugar has on your attitude toward sweet things. You intuitively seek sugar when you need to quiet your physical and emotional pain. You also have the truth of your own pain-numbing experience with ice cream, chocolate, pasta, and French bread. You didn't know it was caused by beta-endorphin, but you sure knew it was happening.

WHY NOT SUGAR?

So why not use sugar as a drug to ease our pain? "It's a food," you say. "What harm can there be in something so natural?" Stay with me, the story is still unfolding.

People with normal body chemistries experience the opioid effect of sugars as simply a pleasant feeling. For sugar-sensitive people, this pleasant feeling can become a euphoria that is powerful enough to create a strong attachment to the food or drink producing the effect. Because we love things that make us feel good, we want more. In fact, this heightened sensitivity to the druglike effects of sugar is the hallmark of the sugar-sensitive person.

Let's review why a sugar-sensitive person has such a powerful response to eating sugars. Remember that sugar-sensitive people have naturally low levels of beta-endorphin and their brains have opened up many more receptors to catch what little beta-endorphin there is. Because of this, sugar-sensitive people will have a heightened response to any substance that causes a release of beta-endorphin. Which is exactly what sugar and alcohol do.

This heightened response happens to Nancy whenever she eats ice cream. Nancy is sugar sensitive. Her natural levels of beta-endorphin are low. Most of the time she feels ugly, unacceptable, alone, and generally out of touch with the world. But when she has ice cream, she feels really, really good. She feels strong, safe, and brave. So whenever Nancy feels upset, she just nestles down with a bowl of ice cream.

As she gets older, Nancy becomes dependent on the ice cream to maintain some semblance of feeling okay. But she is now quite overweight. So she commits to a diet and stops eating ice cream. For a little while she is pleased at her willpower. She starts to lose weight. But she doesn't feel good. She feels morbid, tearful, and hopeless.

Then, right before her period (beta-endorphin levels are at their lowest in women just before menstruation), Nancy starts feeling absolutely *driven* to get ice cream. She is sitting at her desk at work and the idea of chocolate chips and vanilla ice cream grabs her and won't let go. "No, I am on a diet," she tells herself. Nancy goes home. Later her boyfriend calls. She is crabby. They have a fight. She gets into the car and drives to the convenience store at eleven at night. She buys a pint of rocky road ice cream and starts eating it in the car with a plastic spoon she keeps in her glove compartment. She feels much, much better. All is right with the world. For a little while . . . . But as we will see, there will be a big price to pay for the comfort of the rocky road.

Cravings and Relapse

Even aside from the havoc sweets cause with your blood sugar levels, treats like ice cream, candy, and other sugars can create a major problem for the sugar-sensitive person. The drug-induced "happiness" caused by these substances is short-lived and sets up cravings.

As we saw earlier, when you have low levels of serotonin, your brain produces cravings for simple carbohydrates, like sugar, that have the chemical properties needed to move tryptophan into your brain, where it can be used to make more serotonin. In addition, cravings are closely linked to the beta-endorphin system.

Ingesting a small amount of a drug (like sugar) can make a person want more due to a mechanism in the beta-endorphin system called "priming." (*To prime* is to encourage the growth or action of something. You may have heard the expression "to prime the pump," which means to literally pour water into a pump or gasoline into a carburetor to help get it started.) Beta-endorphin priming is the reason it is so hard for a sugar-sensitive person to "just say no" after having a taste of something sweet.

As we have seen, sweet foods or drinks activate a soothing beta-endorphin release. This is why candy is often recommended to alcoholics in early recovery. "It will cut your craving for alcohol," they are told. And that's true. Candy does cut alcohol cravings for the moment, but because it primes the beta-endorphin

system to want more, it sets the person up for even stronger cravings—and alcohol relapse.

Minimizing the priming effect is a key part of stopping cravings. It is also a crucial part of relapse prevention. Priming an
already upregulated beta-endorphin system will have a huge
impact. Remember that after you stop using alcohol or sugar, your
brain will open up even more beta-endorphin receptors to compensate for the reduction in beta-endorphin caused by going off
sugars "cold turkey." Because more receptors are open, an influx of
beta-endorphin triggered by the renewed use of sugar or alcohol
creates a more intense response.

If Nancy stops eating sugar entirely and then one day decides
to have dessert "just this once" at a business luncheon, she will
feel wonderful. With so many receptors already waiting to receive
the big influx of beta-endorphin, she will have an experience of
euphoria that fairly sings to be repeated. If she isn't attentive to
the priming effect of her "just this once" dessert, she may find
herself slipping back into her former big-time use of sugar.

Ice cream and chocolate do produce a wonderful sense of
relaxation, but the sugar-sensitive person can become physically
and emotionally dependent on them. Then they will become
increasingly tolerant to their effects, be driven to eat even more
of them, and experience withdrawal when they try to stop.

This pattern is addiction, plain and simple. Candy and ice
cream are not pleasant and natural foods for the sugar-sensitive
person. Despite the fact that they can help your brain produce
serotonin, they are *not* the solution to either a low serotonin level
or a low beta-endorphin level.

THE SUGAR-SENSITIVE DILEMMA

So what are you to do? You are faced with two powerful dilem-
mas. First, you need simple carbohydrates to get tryptophan into
your brain. Second, your naturally low level of beta-endorphin
gives you a heightened response to things that cause the release of

beta-endorphin—things like ice cream, chocolate, and alcohol. Having these foods makes you feel really good. Eating them actually increases your feelings of self-esteem. But when you eat sweet things (or drink alcohol) regularly, your beta-endorphin system downregulates over time, shutting down many of its receptors in an attempt to stem the influx of sugar-stimulated beta-endorphin and keep things on an even keel, so then you need more sugar to get those good feelings. You end up feeling desperate. It has become even harder to stop because now you have withdrawal symptoms if you do.

Finally you decide to go cold turkey. You stop having alcohol or anything sweet and you weather feeling horrible for the first few weeks. You have managed to quiet the cravings and you feel better. But now your beta-endorphin system upregulates—it opens up more receptors so it can get more beta-endorphin, the influx of which has dropped since you cut out alcohol and sugar. This makes you a sitting duck for relapse. You have lots of receptors sitting there waiting to receive even a little alcohol or sugar and then prime your brain with the message that beta-endorphin feelings are *good* and you should go get some more. If you decide to use sugar or alcohol when you are in this upregulated state, you will feel fantastic since you have lots of receptors to receive the beta-endorphins' "feel-good" message. But when you try to stop again, it will be even more difficult than before because you now have more receptors open and waiting. More receptors mean greater withdrawal symptoms—more receptors screaming when their "drug" isn't there.

It becomes a vicious circle. After what you thought would be just a little bit of sugar or alcohol, your sugar-sensitive brain chemistry starts driving you to relieve the discomfort of these ever-greater withdrawal symptoms. Upregulation explains why we all have huge problems getting "back on track" after a slip in our diet or our sobriety.

If, instead of quitting again, you keep on using a lot of chocolate, sugar, or alcohol, your system will downregulate over time—close down some receptors—and you will have a harder and harder time receiving enough beta-endorphin. In as short a time as a few days, you will find yourself feeling worse. You keep hoping that you can find that wonderful feeling again, but it continues to elude you. You spend your life crawling through the days and trying to keep withdrawal at bay. You end up feeling like a true addict—you can't live *with* your drug and you can't live *without* it. And you think the whole thing is stupid because, after all, for goodness sakes, it's "just" sugar.

BALANCE ONCE AGAIN

The story of sugar sensitivity has given you an explanation for the craziness you are feeling. But now you are ready for a solution. You want to feel better, and medication like antidepressants isn't the answer. *That's not your fault.* This is a story about your biochemistry. And there is an answer.

The solution is almost deceptively simple: if you *eat the right foods at the right times*, you can keep your serotonin and beta-endorphin at their optimal levels. The nutritional solution I will show you is holistic, natural, fun, inexpensive, and easy to learn. What's more, it has no side effects.

Eating the right food is the ideal way to keep your brain chemicals in balance all the time. Making food choices based on an understanding of how your brain and body chemistry work will prevent the dramatic ups and downs in beta-endorphin that lead to upregulation and downregulation, cravings and withdrawal symptoms.

In fact, by adjusting what you eat, you can deal with the three key issues of sugar sensitivity all at once: you can stabilize your blood sugar level; you can boost your serotonin and beta-endorphin levels; and you can minimize the dangerous effects of priming. You don't have to cope with three different treatments, three different dosages, or complex instructions. You don't even have to understand it all.

If you make some simple food changes, your body chemistry and brain chemistry will come into balance. You will reclaim your birthright and feel energetic, optimistic, grounded, competent, easygoing, and connected to others. You will also discover other ways to increase your body's natural production of beta-endorphin without using alcohol or sugar. Exercise, music, good sex, laughter, meditation, prayer, even the smell of an orange—all can evoke beta-endorphin. We'll talk about each of these in later chapters. For now, all you need to remember is that there *is* life after addiction—and it's a very good life indeed.

6

THE FIRST STEP: GETTING STARTED

Now that you have a good sense of the science behind sugar sensitivity, you are ready to put your food plan into action. As you do this, you will be the author of your own healing process. You will use the tools I recommend to make changes in a way that will work for *you*. In my experience, the best preparation for change is to know your personal style. Think about a time when you made a change in your life that really worked for you. How did you approach making that change?

One useful way to discover your style is to think about what you do when taking a trip to your favorite place. Do you just throw a toothbrush and some clean underwear in your bag and head out the door? Or do you go to AAA and get maps and guidebooks, make reservations for every stop along the way, trace your route with a pink marker, pack your bags three nights ahead, and take along your first meal in a cooler? Or perhaps you call your travel agent, who handles it all and hands you an itinerary and your tickets.

Before you read any further, put your finger in the book right at this paragraph, then close your eyes and think about what you would do to get ready for a trip. Tease out whether you like to have a plan or explore things more spontaneously. Whether you need to know all the facts or take things on trust. Whether you prefer to do things all at once or take baby steps so that the process happens slowly.

Whatever you prefer, that's your personal style for making changes in your life. And a crucial part of your success with this program is adapting it to fit your own style. Although this program works much, much better if you take it slowly, it is important for you to start with what you've got—even if it's a preference to do things all at once. Each of you reading this book will go through the process slightly differently.

DON'T USE THE D-WORD

Remember that developing a plan to address your sugar sensitivity isn't about going on a diet—it's about being in relationship with your food and your body. This means that you will have to learn to read your body, to hear what your body is telling you. If you have been feeling "crazy" for a long time, it may seem hard to know what being healthy and balanced feels like. If so, turn to the charts in chapter 3 and read over the words that describe what an optimal level of health feels like. Words like *energy, focus, stability*, and *joy* will help you remember or imagine what is in store for you as you progress.

As you read the next chapters, you will learn what and when to eat to help you reach your goals. You will learn what you like, what triggers you, what makes you feel good, what makes you feel crazy, and what makes you feel clear. This is a *life plan* rather than a diet. You won't get a sheet that tells you in black and white exactly what to do. You will get guidelines and support for making the right choices for yourself. You will continually refine what works for you. Any "slip" you make will simply give you more information about your own vulnerabilities, about which biological system was activated or which brain chemical got out of balance.

When I came back to the program, I read in a newsletter that it was possible to do the first six steps in six months or so, if you stop fussing and fretting and get to work. So I put my head down, focused on one step at a time, and used that as a rough guideline. It gave me a goal—about a month on each step (though step 3 took longer). I was surprised that there was so much to learn about breakfast that it took me a month to get it down :). Especially since I supposedly did it before.

—vbg

For each step, I took the class, joined the list, and tried hard to overcome my shyness and post somewhere every day. I read the books and scoured the website. I bought Kathleen's CDs and listened to them in the car, over and over. I signed up for Ranch, long before it was comfortable for me to do so, and I went. I listened the best I knew how.

It takes what it takes, and this is completely individual, but having a rough timeline worked for me. I was a real mess with not much of a life left, no kids at home, and I was not working, so I made RR my job for six months. About four months after detox, I started to get my life back. Well, the new improved version, with radiance.

—Jeannie

Almost deceptively simple, the food plan you develop will address a number of complex systems all at once. You do not have to master blood sugar and serotonin and beta-endorphin. You simply "do the food" and do the program, and your body handles the rest. As we move through the process, you will also learn how the positive changes you are making affect each of the biochemical imbalances we have looked at. You will try out new behaviors and experience the resulting changes in your body. You will be able to see how these changes are in sync with the science of blood sugar and brain chemistry. Throughout the process, just let your body be your guide.

Now let's get started with your food plan.

TAKE IT ONE STEP AT A TIME

Your sugar-sensitive brain, with its love of impulsivity, may want you to do everything right away. "Give it to me all at once," it says. "Tell me the bottom line. Now!" You want to leap right in and give up alcohol, drugs, sugar, and white flour—even caffeine and nicotine—right now. You want to get on with it.

Before you start, remember two critical points:

☑ Don't try to do it all at once.

☑ Take it in sequence.

Yes, I know I told you to adapt the program to your own style, but these two things are *critical* to your success. Trust me.

First, don't try to do all seven steps all at once! Don't turn to Step 7 and start there. Don't start having a potato tonight. Do one step at a time. Do not proceed to the next step until you have fully mastered the one before it. Each step builds on the last. Don't skip around! The steps are in a specific sequence that will heal your body and brain in a developmental way. The structure and the sequence create something as powerful and as dramatic as the change of food itself.

I used to think my issues were all psychological. I tried all sorts of different pills, therapies, self-affirmations. Anything and everything to deal with my food issues. Nothing worked except this program. I didn't believe it would at first but since I had tried everything else, why not this? What was incredible was that it did work! I kept waiting for the other shoe to drop, thinking that it was just the "honeymoon period" I was in. The honeymoon has lasted for a year and eight months now and continues to blossom and deeply grow. It started so simply with just eating breakfast every day. All you need to do this is to be willing. Because "beginners' mind" was cited so often on the Radiant Recovery community forum, that's how I began. I forgot about everything else I "knew" and put my trust in the program because it worked so well for so many people.

—*Harmony*

There is a whole process for healing addictive behavior embedded in the steps. Healing addiction is key. The change of food heals your biochemistry and the process heals your behavior. If you do the steps as outlined, in sequence, and with enough time to integrate each step before moving on to the next, you will get incredible results.

Many people ignore this advice and do what Tony did. Tony felt terrible when he first came to me. He had been trying to build up his body for six months. He had been going to the gym to lose fat and add muscle. On a typical day, Tony skipped breakfast, then ate an energy bar (a low-fat brand, of course) with an "energy charger" drink for lunch. For dinner he had a large plate of pasta with a huge salad. He drank a pot of coffee each day because it had no calories and gave him energy. In between his so-called meals, Tony snacked on candy for energy. He was exhausted most of the time. His muscles ached and he was on edge throughout the day.

When Tony and I talked, I outlined a plan that included spending a week just doing Step 1 of my program. But Tony wanted more. He left my office and decided he would stop eating sugar and drinking caffeine the next day. And he did. Three days later he had a severe migraine and felt like he had been run over by a ten-ton truck, both of which are signs of sugar and caffeine withdrawal. It was clear to Tony that my program "didn't work."

The truth is, what Tony did doesn't work. If you try to do this program without following the steps in sequence, it won't work. You will feel worse instead of better and you will give up. If you do the steps in the order I recommend, you will stabilize each of the biochemical functions involved in your sugar sensitivity.

As I outline the steps, I will let you know what each one is doing biochemically so everything makes sense. There is plenty of room in the plan for you to exercise your own judgment and make your own choices. But don't tinker with the big plan. Trust that there is a method to this madness. You will get dramatic results if you follow the plan as it's outlined. Done in the order presented, the seven steps and the whole program work.

The food plan I will show you is designed to change your blood chemistry and improve your neurotransmitter function. Even though it may seem obvious and simple, the foods in this plan actually create profound physical and emotional change. Don't be deceived by the simplicity. This is powerful medicine.

> I spent many years bashing myself internally for being so weak that I could not resist ice cream, chocolate, and cake. I did many, many yo-yo diets, and my brain started being less and less effective. I definitely had what you call "mush brain"—and a good bit of anger, too. Thanks for your wonderfully clear explanations of a very complex process and for demystifying things for me.
>
> —*Karen, South Africa*

THE SEVEN STEPS TO FEELING GREAT

Here are the seven steps that will free you from the Dr. Jekyll/ Mr. Hyde syndrome:

1. Eat breakfast with protein.

2. Journal what and when you eat and how you feel.

3. Eat three meals a day with protein.

4. Take the recommended vitamins and have a potato before bed.

5. Shift from "white foods" to "brown foods."

6. Reduce or eliminate sugars.

7. Come alive.

STEP 1: EAT BREAKFAST WITH PROTEIN EVERY DAY

Step 1 is the foundation of your entire program. It starts the process of stabilizing your blood sugar. Many folks think it is a breeze and doesn't require a lot of thought. This, of course, is not true. Mastering breakfast—that is, having it every day, on time, and with enough protein—is actually hard, particularly if you are used to just grabbing a cup of coffee.

Many of the people I work with balk at eating breakfast. "I don't feel hungry in the morning," they say. "Should I eat if I don't feel hungry?" The answer is yes. A normal, chemically balanced body uses hunger as a cue to tell you that it needs more fuel. People who are sugar sensitive usually do not live in a state of chemical balance. Because of this, you don't get the physiological cues to eat that other people do. All bodies need food after a period of fasting, such as the time from dinner to breakfast. If you don't feel hungry in the morning, it's because your "hunger thermostat" is not working properly.

Many sugar-sensitive people love to skip breakfast. Not eating creates a stress in your body, which thinks it is starving because of the long interval without food. So your body releases beta-endorphin that makes you feel lean and mean and focused. This high lasts for a bit until you crash and then are desperate. And if you add caffeine to the mix, it is more intense. Actually eating takes away that rush and makes you feel stuffed. You think you don't like breakfast. So Step 1 may take a little getting used to.

Once you start to eat breakfast regularly, you may start to feel hungry in the morning. This is a good sign. It means your body is starting to regain its chemical balance. You may also find that you feel a whole lot better right away. Many people are amazed at what a difference simply adding breakfast makes to how they feel.

Sometimes people get scared because all sorts of feelings come up for them when they get hungry in the morning. They are afraid that if they are hungry first thing, they will eat, and if they eat, they will gain weight and get (or stay) fat. Not eating allows them to feel safe, in control. When they add breakfast and start to feel hungry in the morning, it threatens their old feeling of safety and they want to quit the whole program.

The important thing is to take it slowly. You don't have to spook yourself. You are simply trying to eat breakfast every day. If breakfast is hard for you, look around and see an interesting type of food you can use to get started on Step 1. "Breakfast" can be as creative as you are. Step 1 has four parts.

Have the right amount of protein for your weight.
Eat within an hour of getting up.
Have a complex carbohydrate.
Have breakfast every day.

Let's take a look at each of these.

Part 1: Have the Right Amount of Protein

To heal your brain and body, you need to eat the right amount of protein for your size. Bigger people need more than little people. But jumping from no breakfast or just coffee for breakfast to a whole big meal takes a little transition. Simply start by getting breakfast every morning within an hour of waking up. Have some protein and a complex carb like whole-grain bread, oatmeal, or a whole-grain bagel. Get into the habit of having breakfast and then take a look at getting the right amount of protein for your body.

To calculate how much protein you need for this step, take your weight in pounds (we'll use 180 as an example). Then you divide that by half (you would get 90) to calculate the total number of grams of protein you want to have each day. Have about a third of that at each meal (about 30 grams, in our example). If you weigh 250 or more, do not go above 42 grams of protein for each meal. If you are pregnant or nursing or engaged in active exercise, you will need to have protein and complex carbohydrate snacks twice a day.

At first blush, this part of Step 1 probably sounds interesting but not really complicated. Let's look deeper. First, it means you have to start connecting with your body: how much do you weigh, for example? You have to know how much you weigh in order to figure out how much protein to have. Many sugar-sensitive people do not really want to know how much they weigh. They hate how much they weigh. It's either too much or too little or if it's a good weight, it might change tomorrow! Right? So having to acknowledge that you weigh this much and therefore you need this much protein can have a huge emotional charge.

Now come some harder things. I say to have enough protein for your body weight. I give you a simple formula. Then come the questions and the struggle. "What do you mean I need 42 grams of protein? How can I possibly eat 42 grams of protein? What do you mean that I need 27 grams of protein? Oh, all right, I'm going to have 16.765 grams of protein and I'm going to count the amount of protein that's in my bacon and the amount of protein that's in this and this and this."

So, embedded in the process of figuring out how much protein for your body is looking at your body or experiencing your body, figuring out how much you weigh, figuring out a mathematical conversion, and then learning about food and how to figure out how much protein is in the foods you eat.

Some people find that very difficult to do. They hate it. They think they have math phobia. And you have to figure out how many grams of protein are in your protein powder or in scrambled eggs. You have to read labels or look things up. For someone just starting, this can be overwhelming. You may ask, "How do I know what to do when I go out to breakfast and there are things that I haven't had before?" "How many grams of protein are in this size sausage thing?" "How can I possibly eat that many eggs?"

Can you start to see the layer after layer after layer of what's involved in doing something that sounds as simple as having breakfast? Going through each of these layers is part of what will heal you. Answering these kinds of questions and confronting your feelings is part of what will heal you. Much of what we do on the online support group for Step 1 is to talk about these kinds of details.

Prepping the oats went well last night, although I put the pan back on the turned-off burner after adding the oats to the pan. I even heard Jo's voice in my head saying, "Don't put the pan back on the burner—it will boil over!" And guess what?! It did! It gave me a good laugh. I guess I'm always testing and needing to learn for myself. Oh well, at least I didn't get mad at myself.

I couldn't wait to peek under the lid this morning! The oats turned out too crunchy for my taste so I added some water and heated them up. They cooked up nicely while I cooked eggs and reheated sausage in the microwave. I added cottage cheese to the oats and ate them with a 1½ eggs/cheese omelet and 1½ pieces of sausage. I got breakfast in just within the hour, but it took me the whole hour in the kitchen. I wasn't as focused as I'd like to be, but, hey, I did it!

Tomorrow I'm going to do the same breakfast just to see if I can do more things ahead of time so I can get the food in me sooner.

—Jane

Let's go back to the practical issue of how to calculate how much protein something has. Read labels. Know that meat, fish, and chicken have about 7 grams of protein per ounce. The protein runs about 25 percent of the total food weight. Protein powders tend to have about 15 to 18 grams of protein per serving. Remember, you are counting the protein grams and not the weight of the food in grams. (If you live in a country that measures food in grams and kilos, it is particularly easy to make the mistake of measuring the weight of your food rather than the grams of protein in the food.)

You also need to learn about dense protein. Dense protein, a term I coined, refers to foods that give you a lot of protein in a normal serving. Meat, fish, poultry, eggs, cheese, and protein powder are examples of dense protein. Milk, yogurt, oatmeal, and bologna are not. Here's why this is important. Let's say you weigh 180 and need about 30 grams of protein at breakfast. You would need to have 4 cups of milk, 6 cups of oatmeal, or 16 slices of bologna. This is not feasible for most of us. But with dense proteins, you could have 2 scoops of protein powder or 4 ounces of hamburger or sliced turkey.

If you are a bigger person and need to eat more than you are used to in order to get the amount of protein you need, you can plan on combining different foods. You might combine eggs, meat, and cheese into an omelet. Or have beans, cheese, and meat in a burrito. Many people on the program find that having a morning shake is the ideal quick and easy way to handle breakfast.

Part 2: Eat Within an Hour of Waking Up

After mastering the amount of protein you need to eat, we come to the part about having breakfast within an hour of waking up. You start having to wrestle with questions, with options. "What do you mean by 'within an hour'?" "What if I wake up to pee?" "What if I get up and let the dog out and I still have my slippers on?" "What if I hit the snooze button sometimes three or four

times, so what is an hour?" "I have to do yoga on an empty stomach for an hour and a half. You don't really mean within an hour
of getting up, do you?" "I have to exercise." "I have to go to the
gym." "I have to get dressed." "How can I do this?" "I have to do
Morning Pages."

All of us in the Radiant Recovery community hear all these
arguments. They feel totally valid to the person trying to sort out
what to do. But underlying these questions is the core issue: "You
can't really mean you want me to change my routine, do you?"
Other people want to know the exact rule so they can go right
up to the edge of it. They want to go into the kitchen and put
something in their mouths 59½ minutes after waking up. They
want to be sure they are following the rule, but just barely. We
may laugh at that, but we know how true it is. It's part of being
sugar sensitive.

This part of completing Step 1 is about understanding the
reason for "within an hour." Why do I say that? It sounds like a
rule, but the process is not about following rules; it's about dealing
with a practical reality. It's about learning to connect with what
your body *needs*, which is to eat in the morning!

I know I've definitely been feeling much more stable
emotionally. I'm dealing with a lot of emotions right now,
but they don't seem to knock me all over the place like
they did before I started eating my breakfasts. I feel them,
then I come right back to center. It's pretty amazing,
actually.

I know personally, I can't even think about weight
loss right now. I have abused my body and soul for most of
my life in pursuit of weight loss and looking perfect. I am
keeping my focus firmly on healing and learning to listen
to my body and feed myself what will help me feel great.
I'm so relieved that all I have to think about right now is
breakfast. When thoughts come into my head about later
steps in the program, I start to freak out, and so I stop and

remind myself that all I'm doing right now is breakfast. I don't have to spend a moment's thought on any of the other steps. Breakfast, I can do.

—*Ramona*

Because you haven't eaten since the night before, your blood sugar is going down and down and down. If you don't intervene, your body is going to start releasing beta-endorphin to soothe the pain of starvation (which is how your body reads the situation) and feel good again. Before you know it, you're going to start having cravings first thing in the morning. Then, POW! You've set off a cycle of addiction without realizing it.

When people say, "But I have to do my yoga before I eat," I ask, "Can you figure out any way to give your body what it needs to keep it healthy and steady and stable?" This shifts you from following a rule to being in relationship with your body. We want to protect your body from the stress of a blood-sugar crash. We also want to help you move away from using "not eating" as a way of feeling beta-endorphin-induced confidence. This is especially tempting when, like many sugar-sensitive people, you usually feel a little—if not a lot—depressed.

I have suffered from depression in the past, the kind where you can hardly move, can't sleep, can't stay awake, can't live, and you feel like nobody loves you and nothing's worth doing. I've had anxiety so bad it kept me housebound. Now I am so mentally healthy I almost don't recognize myself. I wake up cheerful for no special reason. I feel like doing the things I used to enjoy. My mind is clearer. I feel more confident, even at my current weight. I don't fear social events. I don't feel as if the world has me under a microscope. I feel good about the future.

When you're depressed you don't feel like anything is going to help, but just start with Step 1, eating breakfast every morning within an hour of waking up and with enough protein for your body, and see if you don't notice a difference the next day. Some people swear by George's® Shake [a Radiant Recovery® product] for breakfast. Or make some hard-boiled eggs to keep in the fridge. Whatever works is what you do. When you're depressed you have no energy to do much of anything, so find the easy ways to do the program. And remember, we're here for you!

—*Lora*

Part 3: Have a Complex Carb with Your Meal

The next part of Step 1 is to eat some sort of complex carb— something "brown," as I like to say—with your breakfast. Have one serving. The size of the serving will depend on your weight. If you are a little person, have less, like one slice of whole-grain bread. If you are a big person, have more. I do not talk about eating a specific amount of complex carb to balance out the amount of protein you are eating. I don't want you to get caught in the counting game. If you're counting proteins and counting carbs and trying to balance them and making sure you have enough of this and that and the other, you'll get overwhelmed. So I just say have a serving of some good brown stuff. Here are some fun choices for your morning carb:

- Oatmeal
- Brown rice
- Wild rice
- Whole wheat/whole-grain toast
- Potatoes with skin
- Whole spelt/whole-grain tortillas
- Brown rice cakes
- Ryvita crackers
- Whole-grain waffles
- Whole-grain crackers like Wasa
- Whole-grain cereal

- Beans
- Oatmeal pancakes

Part 4: Do It Every Day

Sometimes people laugh at the fourth part of Step 1. But for many of you, doing something every day is really hard. Doing something *every* day trains you to make the behavior habitual. And I mean every day. Not five days a week, or every day but Sunday. You're going to do this every single day so that it becomes an automatic part of who you are. That is training for you. Right off the bat with Step 1, you're learning to do something every day.

Now, what if you have been having breakfast all along? Can you just skip to Step 2? Many people come in and say, "Kathleen, I've been doing Atkins. I know how to do protein for breakfast."

Does that person have Step 1?

No.

Others come in and say, "Kathleen, I've been eating breakfast for twenty years. I'm cool. I know the drill."

Does that person have Step 1?

No.

I usually say, "Can you have a beginner's mind and come to the program as if you did not know how to do it?" Often the response I get is, "Do you mean I have to start eating sugar again?" The answer is no, because that's not what this is about. This is about your relationship to what is embedded in Step 1: getting to know your body and taking care of your body.

That's why everybody does not eat the same breakfast. What Emily has for breakfast will be different from what Rhonda has for breakfast. And what you have for breakfast will be different from what they have. There is no "gray sheet," no "eat this" for induction, the first part of many low-carb diet plans. What is crucial to the process is your having the choice and the skill to say, yes, breakfast, but breakfast for me. This process is about needing to do all four parts of the step, but working out how to do them in a way that's best for you. In this step, as in the other six, you will make the program your own while keeping within the parameters I have given you.

Some Great Breakfast Ideas

You can eat the foods traditionally associated with breakfast, such as eggs, whole-grain cereal, and fruit, or you can experiment with things you may never have thought of as breakfast foods, like burritos, a bowl of soup, a turkey sandwich, or a baked potato. If you still have a problem with the idea of eating first thing in the morning, you can try making a power shake that consists of milk, fruit, oatmeal, and some protein powder. Often this is an easy and manageable beginning for breakfast-haters. If you try this, use either fresh fruit or unsweetened frozen fruit, and choose a protein powder that has no sugars or artificial sweeteners. Most of the people in our community rely on our product, which we call George's® Shake. We have a formula for adults that includes protein, a complex carb, and vitamins. We also have a formula that is just whey protein isolate that is perfect for kids or for adults who love the taste of it.

Most of us use soy milk, oat milk, or almond milk as the liquid for our shakes. And yes, some use old-fashioned cow's milk as well. It is truly a matter of personal taste. I have included a whole set of shake recipes on our website. One important note: don't give children soy milk. It is estrogenic and while very supportive to older women, it is not a good choice for kids.

When it comes to breakfast, don't be afraid to experiment. If your mother told you that you can't possibly have chili or pizza for breakfast, remember that your mother isn't in charge of your meals anymore. If you want chili or pizza for breakfast, and you can get enough protein from it, then eat it and enjoy! You're on your way to creating your own food plan, one that fits your needs today as a unique sugar-sensitive person.

It is really kind of important to remember our protein requirement! It is useful during ALL the steps. That's what's so cool about breakfast. It is like an acorn. It has in it all the elements of the mighty oak that is our recovery.

—*Connie*

Here are some of the things our community members eat for breakfast. They adjust the amounts so they get sufficient protein for their weight. Make up your own list of choices that work for you. Share ideas with your friends. Finding new ideas for breakfast can become an interesting treasure hunt.

- Eggs with sausage, a slice of whole-grain toast, and a piece of fruit
- Oatmeal with George's® Restore (see page 246) protein powder, cream, and strawberries
- Cottage cheese and strawberries
- Corned beef hash with eggs and whole-grain toast
- George's® Original shake (see page 246)
- Breakfast burrito with a whole wheat tortilla, eggs, beans, and cheese
- Chili, cheese, and brown rice
- Scrambled tofu and vegetables
- Whole-grain waffle with George's® Original shake in the batter, and applesauce and yogurt on top

Yes, Step 1 has four parts, four instructions, but the real task is to sort out what those things mean for *you*.

- How much protein do I need?
- What can I eat that will provide it?
- What does an hour mean for me? Is that from opening my eyes, getting out of bed, putting on my slippers?
- What kind of complex carb am I going to eat?
- What am I going to do when I go out for breakfast?

This process is huge. For somebody who is in active sugar addiction, to be able to master it is even more significant.

At first I had to force myself to eat within an hour. I don't even like getting out of bed in the morning, much less doing anything. With the depression, I have to force myself to do everything. Breakfast was just one more chore that was overwhelming. But I considered it like getting out of bed and I made myself do it somehow. Now I'm five weeks into this and I've been faithful every day, I've started to feel better. The depression has shown just an inkling of lifting and, needless to say, I'm thrilled. The only trick I have is the one you showed us, Kathleen: Just do the one thing. Just focus on breakfast. Other than that, it was sheer desperation and forcing myself that kept me going until this point. The hardest thing was not to try to move forward to another step right away.

—Donna

That's the most important thing: if you're starting off, you just do Step 1. You don't worry about what else you're eating. You don't worry about having browns at lunch. You don't worry about the potato. You just do Step 1, because it's really hard. And that's all you need to do. Learn how to master that one step.

This is a key part of the behavioral training that will heal your addictive body and brain. You do not have to do the whole program all at once. In fact, you need to *not* rush ahead. Listen, learn, reflect, build skills.

I guess this kinda comes back to take your time and enjoy the ride. If all we are concerned with is getting to point A, we miss the whole journey of getting there. I am guilty of that. I do that quite a lot with things in my life. I believe that's why time seems to fly by for me—it is going way too fast! When I was building my business,

I kept my looking toward when it would be built, and I missed the whole building-it-up part that could've been fun. I see I am doing the same thing with this program. I keep looking at the day when I will be healed, and I am missing a lot of the journey. I'm glad you brought this up, it makes me aware of it. I need to flow more and find a balance between the two.

— Tom

When I read Tom's post on one of our Radiant Recovery® lists, I asked him if I could quote him because it really touched me. I think he's onto an important issue: we need to spend time in the process of recovery rather than always thinking about getting to the end of it. This means enjoying the art of Step 1 when you are on Step 1. Really learning about breakfast, making things you love to eat, planning breakfast, creating a shake you look forward to having, making a meal that suits you, having it on time, and being able to have it anywhere you might travel are the only parts of the plan you need to focus on now.

Then as you progress, you enjoy—truly enjoy—whatever step you are on. In later steps, this means thinking about journaling rather than planning how to get the sugar out of your diet. Or thinking about eating lunch on time rather than trying to figure out how to have a potato right before bed. This is actually the crux of the program: getting you focused on the solution rather than swirling around in the problem. Doesn't this make sense?

7

THE SECOND STEP: KEEPING A FOOD JOURNAL

The next step in your program to heal your sugar sensitivity is to keep a record of the things you eat and drink and how they make you feel. This record is called a food journal. Before you start to journal, you may hate it. You may continue to struggle with it for a while. And then when you start *using* the journal, you start loving it.

The aspect of healing addictive behavior that's embedded in Step 2 is having a relationship with your body. You don't heal because you obey the "rules" and write in your journal. You heal because writing in your journal gives your body a voice. It allows your body to say, "I like this, I don't like that." Your body speaks to you in the language of symptoms. It doesn't use English. It uses aches and pains and upset stomachs and stiff joints and stomach rumbling and diarrhea and fatigue to tell you very clearly what it feels about what and when you are eating. If you don't write down exactly what your body says, you can't learn its language.

The language your body speaks is very personal. It is unique to you. What a headache means in your body will not be the same thing that a headache means in Vicky's body. So your body will teach you how to understand what it's saying, but you can't learn it unless you're listening. And you can't listen unless you write it down, because you will forget. You absolutely will forget. You'll say, "Oh, yeah, yeah, I got it, I remember." But sugar-sensitive people can barely remember what they ate, let alone how they felt four hours ago.

I've been doing a food journal for years and years, and I still am astounded when I go back and see how clear my body's messages to me are. My body says, *If you do this, that will happen*. If I eat breakfast forty-five minutes late, I will be cranky the next day at 11:00 a.m. even though the content of my meals is perfect. Feeling cranky is my body talking to me in the language of symptoms. It's my body saying, *Feed me on time! If you don't, this is what will happen*. This is why doing a food journal is so very, very powerful.

When women start keeping a food journal, many have to learn how to quiet all the feelings that come up before they can succeed in writing down the details of their food and meal times. Some of what keeping a food journal does is teach you how to recognize your feelings and contain them by stepping back from them a little bit so that you're not awash in emotion. For many men, it's just the opposite. Writing down the data about the food they ate and when they ate it is the easy part. Identifying what they're feeling is difficult. I have noticed through my work with many sugar-sensitive people in the United Kingdom and Scandinavia that feelings are like an unknown and alien language. They simply have less experience in knowing how to describe feelings.

Before I developed the journal format we have now (I'll show it to you shortly) to give people a little structure, some folks would write pages and pages and pages and pages about their feelings. As I was working with them, I'd try to find where they wrote down the food they'd eaten. I'd take a yellow highlighter and mark where the food was—squeezed in among fifteen pages of feelings. Then I'd say,

"Could you write down the food on the left side and the feelings on the right?" And they would begin to see that they had recorded a flood of feelings and only a little bit about the food itself.

As they kept on in the program, they would begin to see that they didn't need to write that much about feelings because their feelings weren't that big anymore. Once they began getting enough protein and eating regularly (see Step 3), they could contain how they felt about their husband or their kids or their dog, because they were simply recording the facts about their no-longer-overwhelmingly-big feelings, not trying to express or process them via their food journal.

If you think keeping a food journal isn't fun, you haven't used it yet. Once you start using it, it is a miracle. The sequence of entries in your food journal over the first three months will be astounding to you. The first entries show you how much chaos and pain you are in. Three months later, when you have been doing Steps 1 and 2, and maybe gone on to Step 3 or even Step 4, your journal entries will show you that because you have kept a record of your food and your feelings, you are now in relationship with your body. You speak its language and you can "read" your own body. Your body doesn't provide a computer printout to tell you what's going on with it, but it gives you clues in the form of symptoms that hint at the bigger picture. These symptoms will be consistent and predictable. You just have to learn to read them.

Your food journal also helps you to understand what your sugar-sensitive body needs and how it reacts to different foods. At this point in the program, you may not know your own eating patterns. You may have nothing more than a general sense of how you feel. You might be able to remember having a good day or a bad day, but not able to be any more detailed than that. Your food journal helps you remember the details of each day. It also provides a baseline for you at the beginning of your program. It gives you a picture of "before." As you continue the program, you will enjoy being able to look back at your journal and see how far you have come.

I love looking back to my very first journal and seeing how far I have come, and how my journaling is so different than it used to be. I have found that I am better able to plan for the things life throws at me. For instance, I know I need to eat more when I am stressed, and this shows up when I travel or get dental work. Or when someone I love moves away. I may not catch it right away, but the more these things happen, the more I learn what I need to do. And now I know what certain messages mean, like a knot in my stomach or loss of appetite or a blood sugar crash during the night. So, yes, I see things and instead of thinking, *What is that about?* I think, *Oooh, I need more food* or, *I need to get back to movement and meditation.*

—*Colette*

STARTING YOUR FIRST FOOD JOURNAL

Begin by getting a blank book to write in. Find a book that you really like, one that fits your style and life rhythms. If you need to carry it with you, get one that fits in your pocket or purse. Go on a hunting expedition to find something perfect for you. Most people in our online community love the journal I designed for the program called *Your Body Speaks*. Also get a pen or pencil you love. Some people like to color in their journals or draw pictures. Molly used colored pens to highlight different foods in her journal. Your journal will tell your story, so enjoy writing it. Don't skip this step. It is really, really important!

Once you have your own book to write in and something you enjoy writing with, keeping a food journal is very simple. First you make four columns.

1. **The date and time of your entry.**

2. **What you just ate or drank.** Include amounts and be as specific as you can. Don't just write "chicken" and "potato." Put

down "one large roasted chicken breast" and "one huge baked potato with 2 tablespoons of sour cream." If you don't know weights or measurements, it will help to learn them. Get a set of measuring cups and spoons. You might even buy a food scale. You don't need to be precise, but your estimates should be in the ballpark. Experiment so that you can begin to estimate reasonably well.

Learn the difference between one cup and two cups of milk, and between four ounces and ten ounces of meat. Reading labels will also give you a sense of the amounts you are eating. Remember to write down what you drink as well. Include things like milk, coffee, soda, juice, or alcohol. Also include the amount of water you drink. Water helps to keep your system clean.

3. **How you feel physically.** Write down anything you notice about how your body feels. Body sensations are physical symptoms. There is a huge range of physical symptoms. They can reflect a state of imbalance or a state of balance. You may not have noticed these symptoms specifically before. The more you pay attention to your body, the more useful your food journal will become. The chart below shows some physical symptoms.

SYMPTOMS OF IMBALANCE	SYMPTOMS OF BALANCE
Headaches	Bright eyes
Stomach pain	Hunger
Muscle cramps	Stamina
Coughing	Natural deep breathing
Fatigue	High energy
Insomnia	Restful sleep
Restlessness	Focus

SYMPTOMS OF IMBALANCE	SYMPTOMS OF BALANCE
Shakiness	Alertness
Muscle weakness	Strength
No concentration	Good attention span
Pallor	Good color

4. **How you feel emotionally.** Pay attention to the nuances of what you are feeling. You may have a hard time with this one at first. Some people write "fine" or "good" for many, many pages. Use the list below to help you learn to describe different kinds of feelings. It will really help you with this step.

SYMPTOMS OF IMBALANCE	SYMPTOMS OF BALANCE
Anxious	Confident
Bored	Excited
Scared	Energized
Mad	Calm
Sad	Happy
Depressed	Interested
Scattered	Focused
Restless	Calm
Irritable	Relaxed
Agitated	Easygoing
Hyper	Patient

Here is an example of what a blank page of a food journal might look like.

DATE & TIME	WHAT I ATE OR DRANK	HOW I FEEL PHYSICALLY	HOW I FEEL EMOTIONALLY

How the Food Journal Works

So go ahead and start your own journal. You can order *Your Body Speaks* from our website (www.radiantrecovery.com), and it will be really, really simple for you to use. Write down what you eat or drink. Try to write it down as soon as you have eaten something rather than wait until the end of the day. Write down your physical or emotional feelings whenever you notice them, not just when you eat. For example, you may find that you feel really energetic at lunchtime, then at 1:30 you feel as if you want to lie down and sleep. Write down what you had for lunch at 12:30 and then write down "Sleepy" at 1:30.

Carry your food journal with you. The more specific and detailed your journal, the more information you will have to work with in creating your own food plan. You may find that getting started with your journal is easy, but continuing is difficult. Sometimes people want to do the program but remain resistant to the idea of keeping a food journal. Often, they have no idea why they are resistant. You may think it's too much trouble or you can't be bothered. You may start with a bang and then fizzle out in a few days: "I didn't remember to take my book with me." "Writing it all down got too bothersome." "I lost it." "I know what I eat, I don't have to write it down."

Oh the journal is key! It always helps guide me on what is missing, and when I don't journal, I start to get sloppy with my food.

—*Heather*

Sometimes we don't want to look at how we eat. Writing things down seems terrifying or petty. You may have feelings of failure or hopelessness attached to the way you eat. Even the idea of a food journal may make you panic. You may be surprised to discover that food has a bigger emotional charge for you than you realized. Or you may have had bad experiences in the past with writing down your food.

Some diet programs require you to keep a log in which you record everything you eat. You are only allowed a certain number of units of bread or meat or fruit, so recording your food becomes a way of seeing whether you have been "bad" and eaten more than you were supposed to. This approach can set you up for a feeling of deprivation and make the food log the target of your frustration or resentment. The log reinforces the negative feelings you may already have about yourself and your relationship to food.

The program I have developed helps you change these old beliefs—and any others that get in the way of making changes in your life. The process is designed to be fun, informative, and free of negative judgments. If negative feelings come up, if you feel bad about writing down that you ate three jelly donuts at 9:00 a.m., remember that you are recording information that will later help you see the connection between what you eat and how you later feel emotionally and physically. That's all. It's not about whether you've been "bad" or "good."

If you find that you keep your food journal for a few days and then forget to do it, write *that* down in your journal. Keep track of whatever comes up for you for *at least a week*. Even if you end up with six pages that say you forgot to notice, keep writing!

A sample page from a beginning food journal follows. Take a look at it to get a sense of what you can put in yours.

DATE & TIME	WHAT I ATE OR DRANK	HOW I FEEL PHYSICALLY	HOW I FEEL EMOTIONALLY
Nov. 10 7:00	2 donuts	Tired	Depressed. Feel like I can hardly function
11:00	2 cups of coffee with cream and sugar	Exhausted	Really good
11:15		Can't stay awake	Crabby about work
1:00	Burrito	Wired	Sad. How can I be wired and sad at the same time?
1:15	Nachos Large Coke	Relaxed	
3:15	2 cups of coffee with cream and sugar	Tense	
5:30	3 beers	Relaxed	Happy

DATE & TIME	WHAT I ATE OR DRANK	HOW I FEEL PHYSICALLY	HOW I FEEL EMOTIONALLY
7:00	3 pieces of chicken Coleslaw Mashed potatoes 2 biscuits with butter and honey	Warm	Satisfied
8:00	Hot fudge sundae with whipped cream and nuts	Full	Feel great!

WHAT TO DO IF YOU DON'T KNOW HOW YOU FEEL

Sometimes you may not know how you feel emotionally. This may be particularly true if you live in a culture where you are told to keep a "stiff upper lip" or "don't air dirty laundry." Trying to differentiate your feelings can feel overwhelming. You may get discouraged because all you are doing is writing "fine" or "okay" or sometimes "horrible" and "discouraged."

Here is a list of words for emotional feelings. Keep it handy so you can use it to be more specific in your food journal.

FEELING GOOD		FEELING NOT SO GOOD	
Able	Grounded	Afraid	Hurt
Alert	Grateful	Ambivalent	Impatient

FEELING GOOD		FEELING NOT SO GOOD	
Animated	Giving	Angry	Imposed upon
Beautiful	Glad	Annoyed	Inadequate
Bold	Happy	Anxious	Infatuated
Blissful	High	Betrayed	Infuriated
Brave	Honored	Bitter	Jealous
Brilliant	Humorous	Blue	Jumpy
Bubbly	Impressed	Bored	Lonely
Buoyant	Inspired	Burdened	Longing
Calm	Joyous	Cheated	Mad
Capable	Loving	Childish	Miserable
Carefree	Open	Combative	Nervous
Caring	Optimistic	Confused	Obsessed
Centered	Patient	Defeated	Outraged
Challenged	Peaceful	Destructive	Overwhelmed
Cheerful	Playful	Disappointed	Panicked
Cherished	Pleasant	Discontented	Petrified
Clean	Pleased	Disorganized	Pressured
Clear	Powerful	Distracted	Rage
Clever	Proud	Distraught	Rejected
Confident	Radiant	Disturbed	Remorse

FEELING GOOD		FEELING NOT SO GOOD	
Connected	Real	Empty	Resilent
Contented	Refreshed	Exasperated	Restless
Delighted	Resilient	Exhausted	Sad
Desirable	Responsible	Explosive	Scared
Determined	Responsive	Flighty	Selfish
Eager	Satisfied	Fearful	Shocked
Enchanted	Secure	Foolish	Shut down
Energetic	Serene	Forgotten	Silent
Energized	Settled	Frantic	Skeptical
Excited	Sexy	Frazzled	Sleepy
Exhilarated	Shining	Frightened	Strange
Expressive	Spiritual	Frustrated	Stupid
Focused	Spontaneous	Grief stricken	Teary
Free	Stable	Guilty	Tempted
Full	Tenacious	Helpless	Tense
Fun	Thrilled	High	Terrible
Generous	Vital	Horrible	Unclear

Go through this list and use a yellow highlighter to mark the emotions that seem to fit your own experience. Recognizing your emotions will get easier as your food changes and your sugar sensitivity begins to heal.

LEARNING TO READ YOUR BODY

At the end of your first week of journal-keeping, take a look at what you've written. *Do not criticize what you ate*. Just look at the facts. You are doing Step 1 and Step 2 now so it doesn't matter if all you ate was a protein-rich breakfast and chocolate, or if you ate ice cream every night at 11:00, or if you skipped lunch and dinner.

Go back to the very first page and look over your entries for the past week. Without judgment, pay attention to what you see. Read what you have written. Try to remember each day and each meal. Don't try to figure out what it means. Don't jump ahead and try to analyze everything.

Now examine the times when you ate. Take a separate piece of paper and write down a summary showing the dates and the times you ate. Don't include what foods you ate or how you felt physically or emotionally. Your summary will look something like this:

10/12

11:00 a.m.	breakfast
3:00 p.m.	snack
6:30 p.m.	dinner
10:30 p.m.	snack

10/13

12:30 p.m.	lunch
2:30 p.m.	snack
8:30 p.m.	dinner
10:00 p.m.	snack
11:00 p.m.	snack

10/14

1:30 p.m.	lunch
3:00 p.m.	beer
6:00 p.m.	drinks
9:00 p.m.	snack

After you have made this summary, answer the questions that follow. Write the answers out. Answer every question carefully. Proceed like a detective on the hunt for information about your sugar-sensitive body.

☐ Do you eat at mealtimes?

☐ Do you eat between meals?

☐ Do you graze throughout the day?

☐ Do you eat at the same times each day?

☐ How long do you wait between meals or snacks?

Write about what you have discovered. Take some time to reflect on your pattern. Let the answer to each of the questions sink in. You will begin to see your patterns of eating. *Don't judge yourself.* The more you are able to just observe and note these things, the easier it will be for you to make changes later. Many people have found that if they write their reflections right in the journal, it becomes fun to go back every three months and see the changes emerging.

I've noticed that lately my relationship with my body has changed some. For instance, before it would tell me *I am hungry,* and I would say, "No, you've already had too much food," and not eat. Now I say, "Oh, you are hungry and you want to eat that? Okay, let's give it a go." And

I am amazed at how darn smart my body is about meal timings and everything. It's like I am tuning in to a sixth sense. I love it!

—*Sandra*

The process of using your journal makes you start thinking about the whole picture rather than just, "Oh my God, do I need to write it to a time schedule, or do I write while I'm eating, and what do I do when I carry it out in public? What happens if somebody looks at it?" What size journal should I have? Do I keep it hidden? Do I take it to church suppers and let people read it and then say, 'Look, here's the page that shows all the feelings'? And what do I do with the old ones?"

Ninety-nine percent of the people who start to journal don't remember that the journal is about relationship to your body. They think it is just a royal pain in the neck. They whine, "Why do I have to do this? Can't I just forget the journal and do the rest?" Then there are the people who use the journal as an excuse to stay stuck for two years. They say, "I can't go on to Step 3, because I can't master the journal. I forget to write in it." And I'll say, "Do Step 3 anyway." What I don't say (but which is true) is this: "You're not ready to be in relationship to your body, so just keep going, and you can come back to the journal later."

How do I know they'll come back to the journal? Because when you get in *relationship* to your body, there is no way that you won't want to journal. It's too much fun. Your body is a wonderful, wonderful source of information—information that no one else in the world can give you. Your therapist can't do it, your body worker can't do it. Your body is the expert on you. She or he has more information to give you about yourself than anyone or anything else in the world.

I love my journal! When I was dealing with a lot of pain and surgery awhile back, it got untidy and my writing looked troubled, distressed. I've discovered that my body *always* knows better than my brain does. It's taught me that if my energy level or circumstances change, I need to adjust my food.

The last third of each page is a review of my day. I might reflect, "Not enough veg at lunch," or "That soup really suited me." I find doing this really soothing. Anything that stands out (like when I started getting obsessive about Ryvita) goes on an "Insights" page. (When I transfer from journal to journal, I transfer the stuff on the Insights page, too. That way all my "Aha!!" bits don't get lost.) I also draw a little cartoon to note that I've done exercise or meditation. Everything has its own area of the page. My journal has evolved quite a bit. Although I always journaled my feelings, before I started the program, I never listened! That's why I do a little reflection *every day* to make sure I'm still listening to myself.

—*Penny*

The challenge of working with your food journal is not *recording* the information. The challenge is being able to understand it. Being connected to your body means learning the language of your physical symptoms and your emotional feelings. You read your journal and you begin to ask yourself, *What's the meaning of this symptom? What's the meaning of this word? How is anger different from rage? How is ecstasy different from joy?*

Sometimes it is hard to look at what the journal shows you. The erratic handwriting. The rage. The righteous indignation. The feeling of blame. The feeling of somebody else did it to you—the feeling of being a victim. You go back and you look at that. *She did this to me.* Or *I can't believe what my boss said.* The munching that happens. When you go back later and look at your journal—even if you didn't write long entries, just making little comments, stuff that's sort of in the margin—you think, Whoa, who is that person? And you remember her. It was you, back then. You remember him, how angry he was or how rigid and tense he was. It was you, back then. Your journal gives you a way to look at yourself over time.

The journal also shows you how things change as you do the food. Another aspect of healing that's embedded in Step 2 is the skill of looking at issues over time. You get to see yourself change before your very eyes. When you get to feeling that your progress is slow, your journal will give you a wonderful reality check.

Don't go to the next step until you love the one you're on. This is a gentle, peaceful process that will amaze you, one step at a time! And unlike any diet you've ever been on, this program gets easier as you go along instead of harder. Each step supports the next.

—*Lora*

8

THE THIRD STEP: THREE MEALS A DAY

I'll be up front with you: mastering Step 3 can be a challenge. It doesn't sound hard at first, but sometimes it takes people months to really get it down. That's okay. Step 3 is about having consistency and stability in what and when you eat. These two traits are alien to the typical sugar-sensitive person, but they are what your body and brain desperately need. Once you have mastered Step 3, you will feel so much better you won't believe it. So let's get started.

Step 3 has three parts:

1. Eat three meals a day.
2. Eat them at regular intervals.
3. Have an adequate amount of protein at each meal.

ADEQUATE PROTEIN AT EACH MEAL

We'll look at the parts of this step one at a time. Let's start with getting adequate protein at each meal, since it's a goal you have a head start on thanks to your mastery of Step 1.

What's the big deal about eating sufficient protein? Protein provides the raw materials to help your sugar-sensitive brain and body heal itself. Most important for you, protein provides the tryptophan your body needs to make serotonin, which keeps you feeling calm, productive, creative, and competent.

Protein also helps to slow down your digestion. Proteins are very, very complex foods, and your body has to work hard to break them down into a simple form that can be utilized as energy. They also help to stabilize your blood sugar levels so you won't have the steep peaks and valleys that are so disastrous for sugar-sensitive people.

Before we go into which foods contain protein, let's take a look at how protein works. Protein is made up of amino acids, which are the building blocks for thousands of cell functions. Your body needs twenty different amino acids to function properly. They are used to make digestive enzymes, to maintain the balance of fluids in your body, to make the antibodies that protect you against disease, to make hormones (such as thyroid and insulin), to build bones and teeth, and to help your eyes respond to light.

Some of these amino acids can be produced in the body. Others, called essential amino acids, must be provided by the food you eat. A food like beef, which contains all the essential amino acids, is called a complete protein. Giving your body complete proteins is important. Eating any type of protein will raise the amount of amino acids in your bloodstream. But in order for these amino acids to actually get into your cells and do their job, you must either eat complete proteins that contain all the essential amino acids or you must make sure that your diet includes "complementary" plant proteins. Let me explain this in a little more detail.

Proteins derived from animal foods (meat, fish, eggs, and dairy products) are complete, while proteins derived from plants (vegetables, beans, and grains) are generally not complete. If you are a vegetarian and choose to eat only plant proteins, it is important to combine them to make sure your body gets all the essential amino acids. For example, rice and beans individually contain incomplete proteins. But if you eat rice *and* beans, the combination provides all the essential amino acids your body needs. You do not need to eat these complementary proteins at the same time. The balance over the entire day is what's important. You can find information about "food combining" in a number of cookbooks and vegetarian books. There are some long-standing myths about the inadequacy of plant proteins and about the need for eating plant proteins that complement each other at the same meal. These beliefs are no longer considered valid. Current thinking suggests that if you are eating enough protein-containing foods and getting an adequate amount of total protein, you are very likely meeting your body's need for complete amino acids.

FOODS WITH PROTEIN

Here are some foods that contain protein.

- **Eggs**
- **Poultry:** Chicken, turkey, game hens, ostrich, pheasant, duck, goose
- **Fish and Seafood:** White-fleshed fish, crab, lobster, clams, tuna, swordfish, cod, salmon, mackerel, trout, and many others
- **Meat:** Beef, pork, veal, lamb, venison, buffalo, rabbit, goat
- **Dairy:** Milk, cheese, yogurt, cottage cheese
- **Beans, Grains, Nuts, and Seeds:** Tofu, tempeh, lentils, kidney beans (and all other beans); quinoa, amaranth, millet, and other grains; peanut butter, almond butter, and any other nut butters; almonds, peanuts, walnuts, sunflower seeds, and other seeds and nuts

The USDA recommended daily allowance (RDA) of protein for a 150-pound adult is 54 grams a day, or a little less than 0.4 grams per pound of body weight. I recommend that sugar-sensitive people on my program eat a little more than that. A good guideline is to have between .4 and .6 grams of protein per pound of body weight depending on your health needs. In the early stages of your recovery, your body may have more repair work to do so you may need to eat more protein. Later, as you feel better, you can reduce the amount a little. This is why I suggest the guideline of .5. You'll recall that this is the amount I recommended in Step 1. So if you learned in Step 1 that you need to eat 30 grams of protein for breakfast, you will also need to eat 30 grams of protein for lunch and again for dinner.

If you have lots of experience weighing and measuring your food, calculating your protein intake may come easy to you. However, trying to measure the weight of food in grams, kilograms, or ounces can be intimidating for some people. Particularly in the early stages of your recovery, you may find it hard to pay attention to this level of detail at every meal. It gets easier with practice. And your history with breakfast is a good foundation for this step.

There seems to be a lot of confusion out there about how to figure out how much "food" you should have to get the number of grams of protein you want for your meal plan. Even though 28 grams equals one ounce, grams of protein do *not* equal ounces of food. Many people have asked for the big secret conversion formula. The big secret is that there is no formula. It's like converting apples to oranges.

A food item (such as steak) is weighed in ounces. Each ounce of that steak contains a certain number of grams of protein. It also contains grams of fat, carbohydrates, and water. (Well, steak doesn't have any carbs, but still.) So, each protein food source "contains" different amounts of protein—measured in grams. Dense protein sources (meat, chicken, fish) contain more grams of protein per ounce than not so dense sources (legumes, nuts, cheese).

The more dense protein sources contain somewhere between 7 and 9 grams of protein in an ounce. So for example, a 3-ounce chicken breast has about 20 grams of protein. But 3 ounces of tofu has only 12 grams of protein. Here is a list of typical protein contents for many of the protein foods you might eat:

- **Meats:** Protein runs about 10 grams per ounce of a standard cut of meat. Ground meat gives about 30 grams of protein in ¼ pound of meat. This is also true for beef, pork, and lamb.
- **Poultry:** Chicken has about 20 grams of protein in a 3-ounce cutlet or about 30 grams in ½ chicken breast.
- **Eggs:** Have 7–9 grams of protein per egg depending on the size.
- **Beans:** Have 8–9 grams of protein per ½ cup, cooked.

You may find it helpful to make a food serving/protein list for yourself with the foods you like to eat and the amounts you'll need to eat at a meal to get sufficient protein. Here is the list Margot made for herself to show some sample protein choices for a meal.

2 eggs and some sausage	4 oz. cottage cheese
2 Tbs. protein powder	1 medium hamburger patty
1 scoop of tuna	8 oz. tofu
1 cup of lentil soup	4 oz. turkey
3 oz. cheese	1 med. chicken breast

Remember, I am trying to have you think about your relationship to food. To do Step 3 successfully, you will have to pay attention to planning your food, purchasing it, preparing it, and eating it. Eating a meal with sufficient protein is very different from "grabbing something" to get by. You will start to understand this the more you work with Step 3. And if this sounds too hard, remember how much better you felt once you were eating breakfast with protein every morning? You'll feel even better having three meals a day with protein.

A Protein That Raises Serotonin

Eating protein causes changes to your brain chemistry. One of the amino acids found in the protein is called tryptophan, and your body uses it to make serotonin, the brain chemical that gives you good impulse control and makes you feel mellow, at peace with the world. As we discussed earlier, if you are sugar sensitive, you most likely have a low level of serotonin. To raise your level of serotonin, you will want to eat foods that are higher in tryptophan.

Below is a list of foods and their levels of tryptophan. You can choose the kind of protein that fits your lifestyle.

PROTEIN FOOD	SERVING	LEVEL OF TRYPTOPHAN (mg)
Chicken (white)	4 oz.	390
Pork loin	4 oz.	390
Cheddar cheese	1 cup	330
Ground beef	4 oz.	320
Tuna	4 oz.	320
Tempeh	4 oz.	310
Cottage cheese	1 cup	300
Tofu	4 oz.	280
Salmon	4 oz.	250
Soy protein powder	1 oz. (2 Tbs.)	220
Scrambled eggs	2	200
Kidney beans	1 cup	180
Quinoa (a grain)	1 cup cooked	170
Almonds	.5 cup	170
Lentils	1 cup cooked	160
Milk	8 oz.	110
Soy milk	8 oz.	110
Yogurt	8 oz.	70

Source: EHSA Food Processor.

This list is just a guideline to help you choose proteins with more tryptophan. Animal proteins are higher in amino acids (and therefore tryptophan) than foods like milk or almonds.

What About Cholesterol?

Although eggs are high in protein, you may feel nervous about eating them because of their high cholesterol. You may have been told to avoid them if your cholesterol count is high. It is true that coronary heart disease correlates to elevated levels of cholesterol in the blood. However, the evidence linking dietary cholesterol (which is found in the food we eat) with the presence of cholesterol in the blood is not so clearly demonstrated.

There is a lot of scientific literature available now about the role of sugar and a rise in insulin levels causing the formation of cholesterol in the blood. Some credible evidence suggests that having a high level of insulin (the hormone that is released when you eat a lot of sugar) has a far greater impact on the formation of cholesterol in the blood than the number of eggs you eat. In fact, a large number of my clients have reported a significant drop in their cholesterol count after minimizing their sugars for six months.

If you normally consume high levels of sugar (including alcohol) and foods made with refined white flour, you will have a high level of insulin. If that's the case, then I do recommend you avoid foods high in dietary cholesterol, like red meat and egg yolks. If you have a cholesterol problem, do some homework. Get as informed as you can about cholesterol. Learn about the different points of view on the best way to reduce your level. If you take medication to reduce your cholesterol, your blood pressure, or your blood sugar, stay in touch with your doctor as you use this food plan. Have your levels checked regularly. All these factors may change as you change the way you eat, and your medication may need to be adjusted.

Why Only Three Meals?

Why do I say to eat three times a day and not six times? Because you have a sugar-sensitive body chemistry, saying no is not your strongest suit. It is very easy to go from having "just a little snack" to grazing throughout the day. You start eating and forget to stop. We are teaching your body how to start and stop. When you end a meal and consciously *stop eating*, you are helping your addictive body to learn healthy new behaviors. You want to learn to start, stop, and wait.

I do not encourage snacking for sugar-sensitive people because all too often snacking can lead to "grazing." Grazing happens when you eat your way through the day. People are often encouraged to eat this way in order to maintain a steady level of sugar in the blood. However, for someone with a sugar-sensitive or addictive body chemistry, snacking can create trouble. Grazing reinforces a lack of impulse control, which is already a problem for people with naturally low serotonin. If they get hungry, they eat right away rather than wait. Learning to start a meal and then *stop* a meal is a very good behavior change for the sugar-sensitive person.

Eat at Regular Intervals

Eating at regular intervals ensures that your blood sugar doesn't drop to a crisis point. If you eat within five to six hours of your previous meal, you are not likely to get into the danger zone. Paying attention to having your meals at regular intervals also helps you pay attention to your food and your body—one of the behavioral goals of the program

Typical mealtimes are 7:00 a.m., noon, and 6:00 p.m.. But your schedule may require something quite different. If you work a night shift or your work keeps you tied up through standard mealtime, you may have to adjust your eating times.

But don't eat breakfast at 6:00 a.m., wait until 2:00 p.m. for lunch, and then eat dinner at 10:00 p.m. If this is your normal pattern, however, and you *know* you won't change it, then you will have to get yourself a healthy snack in between lunch and dinner to prevent your blood sugar from plunging. Carry a snack that includes protein: apples and cheese, nuts and fruit, or peanut butter and a banana, whatever appeals to you. But feed your body more often.

You shouldn't go more than six hours without food except between dinner and breakfast the next morning. Your blood sugar will drop too low and you will become tired, frustrated, and irritable. Your concentration will suffer and so will your work. And if you are pregnant or nursing or working at a high-intensity job, you will need snacks. Simply plan for them.

It may sound as if there is a contradiction here. First I say, "Avoid snacking," then I recommend it. Let me clarify. The best option for sugar-sensitive people is to eat three meals a day at regular intervals without snacks in between. When you eat three regular meals and don't "graze," you teach your addictive body the new behavior of starting and *stopping*. However, I am a practical woman. I know that some people won't be able to eat that way. That's why I present the other option: snacks with protein. It is better for you to know you have another option if you have to use it. This food plan is designed to support you in finding what works *for* you, not in making you work for it.

> Notice that the first five steps are actually adding things
> to your life, not taking anything away.
>
> —*Lora*

If You Have to Eat on the Run

The most important rule for eating on the run is this: *Always plan what and when you are going to eat.* Think through the day before you leave the house. Plan for your danger spots. Take your food with you. Always keep a plastic bag of protein powder with you. Put some in your glove compartment or your briefcase. Carry a knife to deal with apples and cheese. Take your power shake in a thermos or take some of last night's dinner as a cold meal in a container.

Of course, there may be times when you've forgotten to plan and you find yourself in trouble, in which case, go to the second most important rule: *Have a backup plan.* Maybe your backup plan is to go into a convenience store, a grocery store, a deli, or even a fast food restaurant. Know what you can find to eat in those places that you like and that will provide you with protein. Find something good to eat before the candy bar hops into your mouth! Carry the list below with you so you know what to get when you are tired, crabby, or desperate. Think of these as stopgap measures until you can get your real meal. And add your own ideas.

- An apple, two cheese sticks, and a handful of almonds
- A small carton of milk with 2 tablespoons of protein powder
- Cottage cheese and an orange
- Sliced turkey, Swiss cheese, avocado and tomato slices
- Chili in a cup and a baked potato
- A baked potato with broccoli and cheese
- A Caesar salad with extra turkey
- Whole-grain crackers and peanut butter
- A carton of plain yogurt with 10 almonds and ½ cup fresh strawberries
- Two hard-boiled eggs and an orange
- Shredded wheat and milk in a little box, a banana, and a hard-boiled egg
- A breakfast burrito with eggs, beans, and cheese (use a whole-wheat tortilla if you can)
- A turkey sandwich and a pear
- Ricotta cheese and ½ cup strawberries
- A chicken fajita pita
- A veggie sandwich with cheese, avocado, mayonnaise, and mustard on whole-grain bread
- A roast chicken breast with salad

- Spinach salad with tofu chunks
- Egg salad on a whole-grain bagel
- Cream cheese and lox on a whole-grain bagel
- A chicken taco with lettuce, tomatoes, and cheese

JUST DO THREE THINGS

The good news is that to master Step 3, you don't have to make any other changes in your food. You eat three meals a day, you have adequate protein at each meal, and you eat your meals at regular intervals. You don't have to stop eating pasta or chocolate. You don't have to eliminate espresso. Just move whatever you are eating to a mealtime. If you have been going out for ice cream in the evening, you can keep eating the ice cream—just make sure you eat it with a meal. If you have been eating M&M's every day, you can continue to eat them if you like—just eat them with a meal.

You may be wondering how much food you are supposed to eat at your three meals a day. "Where are the tables?" you may ask. "Where are the exchange lists?"

The primary guideline for your meals is the amount of protein. Just as you learned to calculate what you needed for breakfast, you use the same calculation for lunch and dinner. You will sort this out as part of the process. You start with the protein and then add your starch (carbs) and veggies to it. You may still have sweets, just remember to have them with your meal. Or after. After is even better. Don't have dessert first.

Many people get nervous when they aren't told exactly what to do—how many points, calories, or carbs. But if I tell you everything to do, then you are just listening to my instructions rather than trusting your own ability to find what is right for you. Experiment. Try different amounts. You'll find that too little won't work and too much will make you gain weight. *Listen to your body*. Use all that experience you've packed away over the years.

If you have a problem with compulsive eating, if you have an eating disorder like anorexia or bulimia, or if you are currently eating large amounts of sugar and caffeine, your body probably won't know what the right amount is. Simply work with learning to eat three meals a day at regular intervals with the right amount of protein. Work from there. Sometimes this step takes months to master. *That's okay.*

Step 3 has a lot of behavioral healing woven into it. You have to plan, buy, and cook what you're going to eat, then you have to clean up. You have to get enough protein three times a day, day in and day out, You have to get healthy carbs with that protein. You have to do it when you go out to eat and when you are traveling. When you start Step 3, it may feel impossible to master. You think, *Oh my God, what am I going to have? Do I have wheat? Do I have dairy? What kind of fish do I eat? Does it have mercury in it? Do I eat soy? Isn't soy estrogenic?* And so on.

But the process that you learned in Step 1 is embedded in Step 3: if the step is too big, you break it down into little steps. Learning to do that is part of your healing. Remember that the *program* is more than just the food. You are learning healthy behaviors to replace your addictive behaviors. You are learning to say, "This is too much for me to do, I can't do it," and to ask yourself, "So what kinds of options do I have?"

Step 3 also begins the task of specifically healing your sugar addiction by moving your sugars into mealtime. When you have a bowl of ice cream after having eaten a full meal, the effect on your brain chemistry is very different than if you have the ice cream by itself at 9:00 at night. As you move sugar into mealtimes, you start to change the negative physiological impact of your "drug."

Another key part of Step 3, as I explained earlier, is your learning to start eating, stop eating, and then wait until the next meal to eat again. Learning to wait is a crucial part of your recovery. It will serve you well in making many, many behavioral changes.

One of the biggest things that happens when people start

looking at the steps, particularly Step 3, that is they get scared about not having treats when they need them. This is because in our culture, treats represent love. You will think, " Am I going to have to give up my love or my rituals, my ice cream, my reward, my solace?" The answer is absolutely not, but you're going to learn a different way to get these things.

Food is not love. Sweets and treats are not love. They are food.

Love is love. Connection is love. Being with your kids or your pets is love. Reading a good story instead of eating cookies is love. Doing things that you enjoy, making love with some-body that you care about, those are the stuff of connection and love.

This is why I do not want people to rush to Step 6 and go cold turkey off their sugars. It is important to have time to reflect on changing your relationship to sugar. Having sugar with meals creates a steady state rather than intermittent spiking. Having a big hit of sugar from time to time is the very worst thing in the world for addiction. Having sugar with meals starts to create regular intake and regular times. Instead of getting a "hit" from it, you simply have it along with the rest of your food. As that happens, you begin to see that sugar is not love, it is a drug.

And remember that until you get the stability that comes from eating three meals a day with protein at regular intervals and moving your sweets to mealtime, your food plan won't work long-term. Don't be fooled into thinking that this part is so easy you don't have to work on it. If you are sugar sensitive, Step 3 is the key to getting your body chemistry in balance. Give yourself as much time as you need to master it.

I think Step 3 is about learning a set of skills and for some of us that learning can take a long time. I had to learn to plan, to shop, and to cook. It doesn't sound like much, but, I had no idea how to prepare a meal or even what foods make up a real meal. I also had to learn to speak up, to tell others that they might want to work from 11:00 till 6:00 without a break, but that wouldn't work for me because I needed to eat a meal at 12:00 to 12:30. I had to learn how to plan my evenings, how to give up drinking a bottle of wine each evening. Yep, Step 3 took me the longest time.

—*Karen*

9

THE FOURTH STEP: INCREASING YOUR SEROTONIN NATURALLY

Clients often come to me expecting to go home with a long list of supplements to take. They are surprised when I talk about food rather than supplements. People with addictive bodies love to "take something," be it pills, expensive white powder, or special mixtures from a can. "Taking something" becomes the solution rather than creating a lifestyle with a healthy relationship to food. I am careful not to reinforce this mode of thinking. Eating food as your solution to sugar sensitivity demands that you think about what food you will eat, when, how, and with whom. Eating food moves you into the relational aspects of your recovery.

VITAMINS TO READY YOU FOR DETOX

With that said, I also recommend a simple vitamin protocol, because it will speed your body in its return to balance. Vitamin C, vitamin B complex, and zinc are traditionally used in alcohol detox. Since sugar sensitivity is so closely linked to the metabolic pathways of alcoholism, I encourage the use of the same vitamins in this food plan. In the course of this plan, you will be doing a detox yourself. Over time you will be moving away from the more refined foods, reducing your sugar and alcohol intake, and not eating junk food anymore.

Vitamin C speeds detoxification and acts as a scavenger that consumes free radicals, which are the destructive by-products of toxin activity within your body. Vitamin C helps your adrenals recover from adrenal fatigue. Finally, vitamin C helps your brain chemicals work properly by supporting the conversion of the amino acid tryptophan (found in the protein you eat) into serotonin.

The B vitamins are essential in breaking down carbohydrates so the body can burn them as fuel. One of the B vitamins, niacin, is critical to the conversion of tryptophan into serotonin. Many of the other B vitamins do other useful things that I will not go into here. I do not want you to start experimenting with taking lots of separate B vitamins to "maximize" the particular effect you are seeking. This is what addicts do—play around with the variables to get the biggest punch possible. I want to reinforce the holistic approach. So I recommend you take vitamin B complex.

Zinc is a mineral that has a number of beneficial effects in recovery. They are all quite complicated and work at a very subtle level, doing such things as helping insulin do its job and helping digest the food you eat. It isn't necessary for you to know the details. Just trust me when I say that zinc will help your recovery process.

You will need to learn a bit about these vitamins to determine a dosage that fits your needs. I can—and will—tell you what ranges of dosage I have used with my clients, but because there are so many conflicting claims about vitamins, I recommend that you talk to your health practitioner or a person skilled in nutrition about your specific lifestyle and current eating patterns.

An appropriate vitamin C dosage may vary from 500 mg a day to 5,000 mg a day. Doctors skilled in vitamin C supplementation often suggest a "bowel tolerance" dosage. That means starting low and adding a little more vitamin C each day. If you find yourself having gas, diarrhea, or stomach distress, cut your dosage back by 500 mg at a time until the symptoms subside. Vitamins C and B are both water-soluble, so drinking plenty of water will help minimize any overload of these vitamins. What isn't used will simply be washed out of your body.

Always take the B vitamins in a "complex" form so that you get the right proportion of one to the other. Taking the B vitamins in a liquid form will allow you to take the dosage best for you. The liquid form allows you to experiment with different amounts to find what is best for you. Here is one place we will allow your addictive side to have the fun of experimenting with the dosage—within a specifically defined time period. B-complex formulas usually come in a dosage of 25, 50, 75, or 100 mg. Read the label. As we have worked with many people, I have found that a dose of the 25-mg complex is often ideal. If you are in recovery for alcoholism or drug addiction or have a very high-stress job, the 50-mg complex may be better. Do not take more than 50-mg in a given day. And do not take B vitamins at night as they may keep you awake. If you feel at all jittery, take less. It is hard to explain, but when you get the right dosage, you will just feel right. The recommended dosage of zinc is 15 to 25 mg a day. Do not take more than 30 mg in a given day.

As I said earlier, don't take megadose supplements (i.e., vitamins and minerals) or amino acid supplements. This approach reinforces the idea of "taking something" to "fix it," which is precisely the kind of addictive behavior you want to replace: you may have used drugs, alcohol, sugar, or French bread to help you "fix" your "crazy" feelings.

Whether a person is in drug detox, alcohol detox, or sugar detox, their brain is in a vulnerable state during the transition to being drug-free. This compromised state might politely be called "mush brain." In my experience, people in detox can effectively keep no more than three things in mind at the same time. This is why three meals and three vitamins make a good package.

Starting the vitamins now means that come detox time, you will have the skill under your belt. The times of active substance use or substance withdrawal are not the best times to follow a food plan that is complex and requires a huge amount of calculation. You may get to complexity later, but at the beginning, strive for simplicity, simplicity, simplicity. Step 4 is about learning to follow instructions. You simply do what is asked. You do not have to research it, negotiate it, change it, tweak it, or fool around with the concepts. You simply do it.

FINALLY THE POTATO

Now that you have mastered the vitamins, we are going to move on to the flagship of the program—having a potato before bed. Think of the potato as "medicine"—sort of an antidepressant in a brown package. The potato will raise your serotonin levels.

Every night just before bed, have a potato with its skin. Ideally (for biochemical reasons), have it three hours after dinner. This may sound too simple to be part of your healing, but eating the potato will help your body raise your serotonin level and make you feel more confident, competent, creative, and optimistic.

You can eat your potato baked, mashed, roasted, cut into oven fries, or grated into hash browns. Just make sure you cook the potato and eat the skin. You can top it with anything you like *except* foods that contain protein. (If you eat protein along with the potato at bedtime, it will interfere with your serotonin-making process.) Your nightly spud does not have to be a big potato. It can be a russet, a Russian fingerling, or a little red potato. If you have diabetes, do not use a white potato. Use a sweet potato. Experiment. I use a medium Yukon gold with its skin on.

If you find that you are having wild dreams on the nights you have your potato, this is a clue that you have very low serotonin. Eating the nightly potato is giving you a bigger hit of serotonin than you are ready for. You need the serotonin, but it is better to go more slowly. Ease into it and let your brain catch up. Have a smaller potato, or eat just a half or even a third of it. Your body is talking to you. Listen.

I had a spud at dinner, then I had a spud about the size of two hen's eggs (bigger than I usually have) at the three-hour mark after dinner. I went to bed, slept deeply, had some dreams I can't remember, and woke refreshed and with a clear mind, hopeful and purposeful, responsive with a renewed sense of humor, as opposed to vaguely resentful, slightly weary, or burdened. This is delightful!

No, they are not huge differences. They are subtle. How I was feeling this last fortnight is a lot better than what used to be normal. But how I feel today is good. Radiance is a deep thing, not a shallow shine on the surface, it is like a joy which has roots in my being. It's not reliant on day-to-day events and doing.

—*Kath*

Although I said earlier that Step 4 is about following directions, I want to clarify something. The directions are to have it three hours after dinner. But the enjoyment of figuring out how much and what type of potato is one of the places in the program where you get to do individual adaptation. Working with your journal will help you know the difference between eating a big baked russet and a small Yukon gold. As you learn more about what the potato is doing in your brain, you can have fun paying attention and adjusting your potato "dose."

GIVING TRYPTOPHAN A HELPING HAND

Let's talk about what that spud is actually doing and how it can raise your serotonin levels. You learned that serotonin is made from the amino acid tryptophan. Tryptophan comes from the protein you are eating during the day. But having tryptophan available for making serotonin requires more than simply eating foods that contain it. After you eat protein, your body breaks it down into its different amino acids. These amino acids travel to the brain in your bloodstream. They cannot immediately enter your brain cells, however, because there is a blood-brain barrier that controls what gets into your brain cells at any given time.

Tryptophan swims up to the blood-brain barrier with all the other amino acids. But it can't get in right away. There are far fewer tryptophan molecules than other amino acid molecules. It is outnumbered and loses out in the competition to cross the barrier. Think of tryptophan as a runt who gets left behind in the shuffle. This means that even if you eat protein with high levels of tryptophan, that alone won't do the trick. The runt needs help.

Your body has a special way to help the runt get across the blood-brain barrier. When the body releases insulin, the insulin seeks out amino acids to use for building muscle. But insulin isn't interested in the runt. It only wants the big guys. So it carries off the other amino acids to other parts of the body where muscle can be found, leaving little tryptophan behind to hop across the blood-brain barrier and be put to use making serotonin. And more serotonin makes you feel better.

Think about this. If you're eating foods with lots of tryptophan, all you need is a hit of insulin so the tryptophan in your bloodstream can get into your brain to make more serotonin, right? Doesn't this mean you should be eating candy, which will cause more insulin to be released and clear the way for little tryptophan to get into the brain cells? Won't a little candy relieve your depression? Wouldn't you want to be eating lots of chocolate, ice cream, and other sweet things to raise your serotonin level?

This has actually been recommended by a number of professionals in the last few years—despite the fact that it creates tremendous problems for people who are sugar sensitive. "Alter your mood by timing your use of sweets," they say. "Raise serotonin by having jelly beans before you go to bed." " Eat chocolate." In fact, research shows that people who have low levels of serotonin, particularly women who crave carbohydrates, are actually unconsciously trying to self-medicate their depression by eating sweets, white bread, and pasta. But, like other nutritional advice for people with normal body chemistries, the advice to eat chocolate is not good for people who are sugar sensitive. For you—and others with your special body chemistry—raising your insulin level by eating carbohydrates like jelly beans, chocolate, or French bread creates even more trouble.

> "How do you force the will?" What converted me totally to the steps and made me trust it absolutely was the realization that for me, will had NOTHING to do with it. I had been born with fierce willpower and am stubborn as a mule, but that did nothing to heal my biochemistry. But I came into my steps with that same mind-set. I had difficulties, and my moment of insight came when I stopped trying to intellectualize it and said out loud "I give up" and just did it.
>
> I healed because the steps did it. Well, my own desire for things didn't go with Step 3. In fact, I wasn't planning to give coffee up at all :-) Or my weekend wine for that matter! But—my Step 4 did it for me. Once I wasn't working against my biochemistry but healing it, it happened on its own. No will. No willpower. Not even much effort. I thought that was impossible.
>
> —Mosaic

Foods like these can send the level of sugar in your blood sky high and set you up for a huge crash. True, you will get more than enough insulin to help little tryptophan cross the blood-brain barrier, but you will also get a blood sugar spike and plunge. In addition, sweet foods will cause a big release of beta-endorphin, and that will prime your brain to crave even more sugar. Remember, we are trying to quiet the priming effect.

Since all carbohydrates raise your level of insulin, there are other ways to get tryptophan into your brain cells to make serotonin without the harmful effects of jelly beans or French bread. Complex carbohydrates like baked potatoes, whole-grain breads, and brown rice will give you a slow and gradual insulin response, not a blood sugar spike. Those baked potatoes with their skins on seem to work really well. Baked potatoes have a high level of potassium. Potassium is what is called a cofactor for insulin, and gives the potato a potent effect.

Not only do potatoes give you a rise in insulin, they seem to offer emotional comfort as well. One scientific study (S. Holt et al.) measured the "satiety index" of common foods. This index gave a value to how full certain foods made people feel after eating them. Here are a few of the foods they measured:

FOOD	SATIETY INDEX
Potatoes	323
Whole-grain bread	157
Popcorn	154
Rice	138
Crackers	127
Cookies	120
Pasta	119
Jelly beans	118
Cornflakes	118
French fries	116
White bread	100
Ice cream	96
Chips	91
Doughnuts	68
Cake	65
Croissant	47

Mr. Spud is clearly the winner! Scientific investigation corroborated what all the sugar-sensitive people have been reporting. And eating potatoes is not only satisfying, it actually changes your brain chemistry.

10

THE FIFTH STEP: GOING FROM WHITE TO BROWN

Congratulations! Now that you have completed Steps 1 through 4, you are ready for Step 5, the shift from "white foods" to "brown foods." In this step you start adjusting the kinds of carbohydrates you are eating. It is the easiest of all the steps. In fact, you started to ease into Step 5 when you did Step 1 and added the complex carbohydrate to breakfast. Sometimes by the time a person gets to Step 5, it is a total nonissue. For others of you, Step 5 may be harder because of your love affair with carbs. Carbohydrates include some alcoholic beverages (beer, wine, and drinks mixed with fruit juice), sugars including sucrose (table sugar), fructose (fruit sugar), lactose (milk sugar) and a few others, and starches like bread, pasta, cereal, vegetables, beans, and grains.

Carbohydrates can be simple, like beer, wine, and the sugars; or complex, like the starch found in brown rice or vegetables. Whether a carbohydrate is simple or complex depends on how many molecules it has. While sugars are considered simple carbohydrates, starches are complex carbohydrates because they consist of three or more sugars joined together to make a long chain of molecules. Starches come from grains (wheat, corn, rice, etc.), beans (peas, lentils, chick peas, etc.), and tubers (potatoes, yams, etc.).

Why do we care whether the carbohydrates we eat are simple or complex? Because in order for carbohydrates to be converted into fuel that your body can burn, their molecule chains must be short enough to go through the wall of your stomach or small intestine and get absorbed into your bloodstream. Before this can happen, your body has to digest the complex carbohydrates you have eaten, breaking them down into simpler forms. In fact, your body eventually breaks down all carbohydrates, even things like broccoli, into the simplest form of sugar, called glucose.

When we talk about your blood sugar level, what we are actually talking about is the amount of glucose in your blood. Remember that sugar is not bad. In fact, it is life-giving. But we want you to have all the positive effects of sugar in your body without the negative effects. To prevent your sugar-sensitive body from getting too big a rush of sugar and sending your blood sugar skyrocketing (and later plummeting), you want to slow down the release of sugar into your bloodstream. You also want to avoid the beta-endorphin priming that comes with having alcohol or simple sugars. Avoiding simple carbohydrates, which are absorbed into your bloodstream quickly, and eating more complex carbohydrates, which are absorbed slowly, can help do this.

I have just started eating more brown rice (after a lifetime of really not liking rice), and I've had blue corn chips too. I've had quinoa and barley, but only occasionally, like once each in recent memory. Teff (an ancient grain) and amaranth I haven't really had. Hmmm, not much of a grain person . . . I like tortillas and bread. They can be sprouted wheat tortillas and whole-grain chewy bread . . . but I don't have a lot of interest in a pile of quinoa on the plate. I guess that's why I'm here, though, to push that envelope!

—*Rebecca*

In addition, certain carbohydrates like whole grains and vegetables contain fibers that are difficult for your body to break down. Fibers are made from long chains of glucose that are joined together as either cellulose or pectin. Your body cannot digest cellulose fibers, like bran, so they provide bulk but little nutritional value. Pectin fibers, found in apples, oats, and beans, are water-soluble and can be digested. Water-soluble fibers are great allies for sugar-sensitive people because your body takes longer to break down their long chains of molecules. The small intestine has to work hard to get the glucose out. This takes time and creates a slow, stable, steady stream of glucose into your blood. For example, brown whole-grain bread is "slower" than French bread to break down because the brown part is the fiber.

THE CARBOHYDRATE CONTINUUM

In Step 5 of your food plan, you will start to shift your carbohydrate intake away from the quickly digested simple carbohydrates to the slower, more complex ones. You will eat fewer foods made with white flour and start eating more whole-grains and foods with soluble fiber.

The carbohydrate continuum on the next page shows the relative complexity of different carbohydrates. To the left are carbohydrates that are absorbed most quickly into your bloodstream. To the right are carbohydrates that contain a lot of soluble fiber and are absorbed more slowly.

This chart gives you general guidelines, but remember that a certain food may be slower or faster to break down depending upon how it's prepared. Digesting a baked potato with skin takes longer than digesting skin-free mashed potatoes because the brown skin of the potato contains fiber. Digesting cooked broccoli is faster than digesting raw broccoli because the cooking breaks down the fiber before you eat it. Your body has to do less work.

When you design your food plan, you will want to include a good supply of complex carbohydrates. Choose the slowest ones.

THE CARBOHYDRATE CONTINUUM

ALCOHOL	SIMPLE SUGARS	SIMPLE STARCH	COMPLEX STARCHES	COMPLEX STARCHES	WOOD
beer wine	glucose sucrose fructose white sugar honey corn syrup all the others	**"white things"** white flour products white rice pasta	**"brown things"** whole grains beans potatoes roots	**"green things"** broccoli and other green vegetables **"yellow things"** squash and other yellow vegetables	not digestible

Your body eventually breaks all carbohydrates down to glucose. How quickly your body can do this depends on how complex the food is. The foods on the left of the continuum are very simple with only a few molecules. They are absorbed rapidly. The foods on the right of the continuum are very complex and require the body to work hard to break them down. This takes a long time and means that you will not get a sugar high from broccoli!

Learn to use the carbohydrate continuum. Start moving from "white things" to "brown things" and "green things" on the carbohydrate continuum.

Now let's take a look at the continuum in more detail.

Alcohol

Alcohol is made from adding yeast to certain foodstuffs in order to ferment them. Wine is made from fermenting grapes or other fruits, beer is made from fermenting grain, and hard liquor is made from first fermenting grain and then distilling the ferment to make it more concentrated. So beer and wine contain a high level of fructose (a simple sugar) and alcohol, which can be absorbed directly from the stomach and requires no digestion at all. Hard liquor does not contain carbohydrates because it is a distillate of the carbohydrate base from which it is made. However, if it is mixed with fruit juice, it becomes even more potent for you. The result is that drinking alcoholic beverages is going to have a nearly immediate (and devastating) effect on your blood sugar level as well as causing beta-endorphin priming.

Simple Sugars

The list below will give you a sense of how many foods contain sugar. Most people have no idea that sugar comes in so many forms. The sugars in bold print are overt sugars. These are the sugars that most people know about and use. Remember, though, that everything on this list is a sugar.

agave	**brown sugar**
amazake	cane juice
barley malt	**confectioners' sugar**
beet sugar	**corn syrup**
brown rice syrup	corn sweetener

date sugar

dextrin

dextrose

fructose oligosaccharides

fructose

fruit juice concentrate

galactose

glucose

granulated sugar

high-fructose corn syrup

honey

invert sugar

lactose

maltodextrin

malted barley

maltose

mannitol, sorbitol, xylitol, maltitol

maple sugar

microcrystalline cellulose

molasses

polydextrose

powdered sugar

raisin juice

raisin syrup

raw sugar

Sucanat

sucrose

sugarcane

turbinado sugar

unrefined sugar

white sugar

Sugars are found in an extraordinary variety of foods. Most of us recognize that things like candy bars, cake, cookies, sweetened cereals, chocolate milk, soda, or ice cream contain sugars. But few people realize how many other foods contain hidden sugars. Canned ravioli, Slim-Fast, nutritional bars, prepared meat loaf dinners, and dried fruit can contain more sugars than you might expect.

I classify sugars as either overt (the ones that are obviously sugars) or covert (the ones that are hidden). Let's take a look at the sugar content of some of the foods you might be eating regularly—these are what I class as overt sugar foods. I have calculated the impact value for each of these overt sugars by determining the density of the sugars and fiber in proportion to the total carbohydrate and then factoring in the portion size. *The higher the impact, the more intense the sugar "hit."* I have ranked them according to their impact value.

FOOD	SERVING SIZE	GRAMS OF SUGARS	IMPACT
Ice cream Blizzard	1	88	**72.08**
M&M's	5-oz. package	82	**64.04**
McD's chocolate shake	16 oz.	58	**53.16**
Ice cream	8 oz. (½ pint)	45	**44.68**
Coca-Cola	12 oz. can	39	**39.02**
Kool-Aid	12 oz.	38	**37.50**
Chocolate chips	½ cup	43	**33.25**
Chocolate cake with icing	1 piece	31	**26.31**
Frozen yogurt, soft-serve	1 cup	32	**24.38**
Butterfinger candy	2.16 oz.	30	**20.97**
Jell-O Pudding Snack	1	23	**18.89**
Maple syrup (Hungry Jack)	3 oz.	30	**18.39**
Chocolate milk	8 oz.	20	**15.72**
Jell-O Snack	1	18	**18.00**
White sugar	2 packets	16	**11.99**
Gum	1 stick	2	**.67**

Source: EHSA Food Processor. Impact score by DesMaisons

The typical dose of sugars one might receive in manufactured foods runs about 35–40 grams per serving. If you start to read labels, you will be surprised to see how consistent this level of sugar is. Observe your own response to the "taste" of sweet foods. Usually we have come to expect that this level of sugar tastes "right." Sugar-sensitive people tend to be more comfortable with sweeter foods.

Fruits and fruit juices are also high in sugars. Most people assume that the sugars found in fruit are very healthy because they are "natural." It is true that fruits contain vitamins not found in things like Coca-Cola. However, your sugar-sensitive body registers the sugar in fruit and responds to it as powerfully as the sugar in chocolate chips. Fruit juice in particular is a sugar with a high impact value because it has very little fiber to slow it down. Let's take a look at the sugar content of some fruit juices. I have used a 12-ounce serving size so you can compare the sugar content of a fruit juice to that in a 12-ounce can of soda, which usually has about 38 grams of sugar. The juices highest in sugar are at the top.

JUICE	SERVING SIZE	GRAMS OF SUGAR
Grape juice	12 oz.	54
Apple juice	12 oz.	41
Orange juice	12 oz.	38
Grapefruit juice	12 oz.	27
Tomato juice	12 oz.	08

Source: EHSA Food Processor.

Although drinking orange juice instead of cola is more nutritious, the sugar content is almost exactly the same. Also, notice how much more sugar grape juice contains. This is why concentrated grape juice is so often used as a sweetener in "natural" foods. People think that grape juice is healthier than refined white sugar. But your response to a certain food is determined by the intensity of the sugar "hit." One broadly marketed health juice drink made as a "vitamin and herbal fortified drink for women" has 72 grams of carbohydrate, of which they say 56 grams are sugars and 5 grams are fiber. It is not clear what the remaining 11 grams are. But at any rate, many sugar-sensitive people will be drawn to this "fortified" drink because it appears so "healthy." By now, you can well see why such a drink would make you feel really high in the short run.

Let's take a look now at the sugar in whole fruits, with those highest in sugar at the top (see table on opposite page).

If you compare the values of these fruits to the foods in the chart for overt sugars, you will start to see why making some small changes in what you eat—like eating berries instead of applesauce or raisins—can have a huge effect on how you feel.

These charts show you how to identify the overt sugars in your diet. Start noticing how often you have sugar foods. Mark the sugar foods in your food journal. Don't get discouraged if you find that a significant proportion of what you eat is high in sugar. Don't stop eating sugar foods yet, but start being attentive. If you have something sweet, plan to have it with your meals so that you temper the impact of the sugar with the other foods you are eating. Start cutting down on the overt sugars as best you can. But don't scare yourself. Remember, this plan is not about deprivation. It's about paying attention and making informed choices. The more you understand how all of this fits together and the more you understand the equation of your own body, the better you will be able to make choices that work for you.

Think about ways you can creatively have the sweet foods that you like. Have whole fruit (with fiber) instead of juice. Substitute juice for soda because it is more nutritious but dilute the juice so you won't get a huge sugar hit. For example, if you make a juice spritzer out of 3 ounces of orange juice with 9 ounces of sparkling water instead of having a can of soda, you can reduce

FOOD	SERVING SIZE	GRAMS OF CARBS	GRAMS OF SUGARS	GRAMS OF FIBER	IMPACT
Applesauce, sweetened	1 cup	50.75	47.66	3.06	**41.89**
Raisins	1 box (1.5 oz)	34.01	32.29	1.72	**29.03**
Grapes	1 cup	24.48	27.52	1.60	**25.05**
Dried apricots	½ cup	50.22	33.44	4.18	**19.48**
Apple with peel	1 large	32.44	25.44	5.72	**15.46**
Banana	1 medium	27.61	21.82	2.83	**15.00**
Orange	1 large	21.71	17.30	4.42	**10.26**
Pear	1 medium	25.07	17.50	3.98	**9.43**
Blueberries	½ cup	10.22	8.27	1.96	**5.10**
Strawberries	½ cup	5.05	4.06	1.66	**1.93**
Apricots	1	3.89	3.05	.84	**1.73**
Raspberries	½ cup	7.13	5.84	4.18	**1.36**

Source: EHSA Food Processor. Impact score by DesMaisons

your sugar intake drastically. If you have been drinking four sodas a day, you will cut your sugar intake by 112 grams every day!

My clients frequently ask me about the advisability of using "sugar-free" products. There are two parts to the answer. Many products advertised as "sugar-free" simply mean they are free from *certain kinds* of sugars. If a manufacturer uses a trisaccharide (a sugar with three parts in it), it does not have to be called a sugar since legally it is a starch. Maltodextrin falls into this category. You will respond to maltodextrin as if it is a sugar.

Other sugar-free products use aspartame (NutraSweet) as a sweetener. Aspartame is made from phenylalanine, which is an amino acid. High doses of any single amino acid can throw off the balance of aminos in your brain and body. Since phenylalanine is a precursor to dopamine and norepinephrine, which are both stimulating neurotransmitters, high usage of NutraSweet can create an "upper"-like effect. You may find that you really like the effect you get from sugar-free products. I encourage my clients to stay away from products with aspartame both for their addictive potential and because they reinforce the dependence upon sweet taste. This is one more place you will want to make choices about what is right for you.

Many people have switched from ice cream to low-fat frozen yogurt as a way to reduce calories. Low-fat frozen yogurt has fewer calories from fat but far more sugar. A sugar-sensitive person does better with real ice cream because the fat it contains actually slows the speed at which the sugar is absorbed into your bloodstream. Now, I am not advocating the long-term use of ice cream, but if you do eat these desserts, you might experiment to see whether ice cream or fat-free frozen yogurt affects you differently.

Your goal right now is to start paying attention to the overt sugars. I will speak more about the covert sugars later on. In the meantime, do what you can to reduce your overt sugar levels.

"White Things"

The carbohydrate continuum chart will help you see the relationship of sugar and what I call "white things," "brown things," and "green things." I use these terms because it is easy to remember these simple images as you make your own food choices. Just as you have begun to notice the sugars, I now want you to look at the simple starches in your diet. I use the term "white things" to identify those starches that are refined. The term is apt because these "white things" have literally had the brown part of the grain removed to make them more visually attractive. Taking out the brown part also makes them sweeter because it takes less time for your body to digest the starch and convert it to sugar.

Here are some examples of "white things":

Bagels	Noodles
White bread	Pancakes made with
Cake	white flour
Cereal	Pasta
Cookies	Pastry
Crackers	Pie
Croissants	Waffles
Flour tortillas	White rice
Macaroni	

The chart that follows shows you the amount of carbohydrate, the amount of sugar, and the amount of fiber for various "white things," with those highest in sugar at the top. It also includes the impact value. It will give you a clear sense of how the level of fiber in a food can slow the impact of the sugar. Compare the impact values of these foods to the foods in the overt sugar list.

These are considered "typical" servings in the nutrition tables. You may eat a bigger slice of pie than two inches or more than half a cup of rice. Adjust the comparisons according to the size of the serving you eat. If you have two cups of Raisin Bran for breakfast, you will have more than twice the sugar in a sugar donut. So you can see why it is important to start reading labels.

You may look at this chart and say, "Well now, which is the 'best' white thing for me to eat?" And you can see that a bagel is better than white bread because it has a little more fiber. But wait before choosing the best white thing. Look at the list of "brown

A COMPARISON OF "WHITE THINGS"

WHITE THING	SERVING	TOTAL CARBS (GRAMS)	SUGAR (GRAMS)	FIBER (GRAMS)	IMPACT
Donut, powdered sugar	1	24.0	12	1.0	5.5
Corn bread (KFC)	1	25.0	10	1.0	3.6
Raisin bran cereal (Kellogg's)	1 cup	42.9	15	7.0	2.7
Plain pancakes (4" each)	3	41.8	10	9.0	1.8
Blueberry muffin	1	27.3	6	1.0	.88
Rice Krispies cereal (Kellogg's)	1 cup	22.8	2	0.3	.21
Bread (firm white)	1 slice	33.2	3	1.5	.08
Corn flakes cereal (Kellogg's)	1 cup	21.6	2	0.7	.08

WHITE THING	SERVING	TOTAL CARBS (GRAMS)	SUGAR (GRAMS)	FIBER (GRAMS)	IMPACT
Bread (soft white)	1 slice	28.6	2.2	1.2	.08
English muffin	2	52.0	3.9	3.0	.07
Crackers (Ritz)	8	14.6	1.2	.38	.07
Croissant	1	26.1	1.8	1.5	.03
White rice (cooked)	1 cup	44.6	.32	.63	.00
Crackers (saltines)	8 crackers	17.2	.36	.72	–.01
Pita bread (6½" diameter)	1	33.4	.78	1.32	–.01
Bagel	1	37.9	1.07	1.63	–.02
Flour tortillas (10" round)	1	40.3	.87	2.38	–.03
Spaghetti (cooked)	2 cups	79.2	3.64	7.56	–.18

Source: EHSA Food Processor. Impact score by DesMaisons

things" that follows, and you will begin to see the dramatic difference between white things and brown things.

Most commercially sold bread contains refined white flour even though it is labeled as "brown" or "whole-grain." For example, breads with "wheat flour" or "flour" at the head of their ingredients lists are still made with refined white flour. Unless the first ingredient says "whole wheat flour," think of it as a "white thing." Also check the food label for the amount of fiber. Look for 2 or more grams of fiber in each serving. You can see that white things are "white" because they don't have much fiber. Remember, the higher the fiber, the longer it will take to digest, and the slower the flow of sugar into your bloodstream will be.

Look at the fiber values for white things and compare them to the fiber in the chart of brown things below. There is a big difference. Whole grains have far more nutritional value because the "brown stuff" in whole grains is what has the vitamins in it.

Take a page in your food journal now to make a list of the things you eat that have white flour in them. Your goal is going to be to shift your intake of white things to brown things. For many of these foods, you can substitute whole-grain products such as 100 percent whole wheat bread or whole wheat pasta. You can have brown rice instead of white rice. You can try shredded wheat instead of Rice Krispies. Or you can have oatmeal, which is the best of all because so much of its fiber is soluble. Whole-grain foods are more complex and give your body a solid, consistent fuel to draw from. The lower the impact score, the better.

When you first looked at the list of white things, were you surprised to see how many of the foods you love were there? Sugar-sensitive people *love* white things—sometimes even more than ice cream or other sweet treats. It might spook you to think of not eating white things. Some people love breads more than anything. If so, be gentle with yourself. No one is going to take away your favorite foods. The idea is for you to move toward using more complex carbohydrates *as you can*. Maybe you can start by finding a new bread that is a little heartier than the one you eat now. Check out the cereal options. Be careful to read labels, though. Often foods

CEREAL	IMPACT
All-Bran (Kellogg's)	−3.08
Oatmeal/porridge (unsweetened)	−0.11
Grape-Nuts (Post)	−0.06
Cheerios (General Mills)	−0.05
Shredded Wheat (Post)	0.00
Corn Flakes (Kellogg's)	0.08
Rice Krispies (Kellogg's)	0.20
Raisin Bran (General Mills)	2.67
Oatmeal (cinnamon/spice)	5.70
Cap'n Crunch (Quaker Oats)	6.19
Frosted Flakes (Kellogg's)	6.50

are labeled "all natural" and they look "brown" but they are filled with sugars. Commercially made granola is often like this. It sure *looks* good for you, but it has grams and grams of sugar.

If you find that giving up white things is difficult, do what you did with the sugars. Try not to eat them alone. Have your white thing with some other slow food. Make change at the pace that works for you. You do not have to hurry this process. We are looking for solid long-term success, not dramatic short-term results.

When you do eat on the "brown" and "green" side of the carbohydrate continuum rather than the "white" side, you'll start noticing big changes in your sense of well-being and your energy level. When you look at your food journal you will see the connection between your new way of eating and your feelings.

You may find that this step is hard. We love white things. They often represent comfort and love. Many people would kill for French bread. Notice your own emotional attachment to white things. See if you can tease out what part of your enjoyment of white things comes from the biochemical response they give you and what part of your enjoyment comes from your emotional association with what you are eating.

For example, sugar cookies in the shape of Christmas trees covered in green icing have a huge association for me with the joy of Christmas time. I used to find it very hard to even think about not eating them at Christmastime. The idea of giving them up, even if I were pondering it in July, made me so sad and angry about having such a stupid body chemistry that I would go eat something sweet to comfort myself!

I had to learn to be patient with myself and understand the full emotional impact of those cookies. I found that the feelings I associated with Christmas tree cookies were really about being cared for at Christmas. It seemed as if all the other children had mothers who made them cookies at Christmas. My mother worked, so we rarely got homemade cookies. When my children were little, I started making them iced green Christmas trees as a way to show them the love I had wanted when I was little. Once I realized this, I gave myself permission to have some cookies at Christmas, but I also paid attention to the bigger picture of all the white things that are associated with holidays and showing love. I chose to eat a few cookies because they seemed the most important emotionally. But I didn't eat the pies and the cakes and the sweet breads. I learned to recognize the many emotional issues wrapped up in the foods I wanted and to make choices that would support my food plan. Now I don't even crave the Christmas tree cookies. (But I still make them and give them to my friends who aren't sugar sensitive.)

The bottom line for Step 5 is, do what you can to shift your carbohydrate intake from white things to brown things. But do it at the rate you feel comfortable with.

"Brown Things"

"Brown things" include foods higher in fiber, such as whole grains, seeds, and beans. This list shows examples of what I call "brown things."

Whole-grain bread
Whole-grain cereal
Whole-grain pasta
Whole-grain pancakes
Whole-grain tortillas (corn or whole wheat)
Granola, no sugar added
Brown rice
Oatmeal
Potatoes with skin
Kidney beans (used in chili)
Black beans
Garbanzo beans (chickpeas)
Hummus
Lentils
Millet
Quinoa
Soy beans
Polenta
Sweet potatoes

Brown things are an excellent source of complex carbohydrates. You might recognize some of these foods from the protein chart. Beans and grains contain both protein and carbohydrate. Grains can have as much as 24 percent of their cooked weight as carbohydrate and as little as 3 percent as protein, while beans can have 19 percent of their weight as carbohydrates and 8 percent as protein. Brown things provide your body with solid nourishment and sustained energy. They will help you maintain a steady blood sugar level and support the optimal-level feelings we talked about in chapter 3. Here again is the chart showing the difference in your feelings between times when your blood sugar is at an optimal level and when it has plummeted as a result of eating sugars and foods made with refined flour. These are just a few of the many benefits of shifting from white things to brown things.

OPTIMAL BLOOD SUGAR	LOW BLOOD SUGAR
Energetic	Tired all the time
Tired when appropriate	Tired for no reason
Focused and relaxed	Restless, can't keep still
Clear	Confused
Good memory	Trouble remembering things
Able to concentrate	Trouble concentrating
Able to problem-solve effectively	Easily frustrated
Easygoing	More irritable than usual

The chart on page 168 will show you the sugar in various brown things. All servings in this chart reflect $1/2$ cup of cooked (in most cases this means boiled) food.

Compare the foods in this chart to those on the white things list. The higher levels of fiber in the brown things is what slows the sugar absorption down and keeps your blood sugar and brain chemicals at optimal levels.

As you add brown things into your diet, keep noticing how you respond to what you are eating. If you find yourself becoming really attached to a given food, try to sort out what is going on. Anne Marie developed a recipe for a pumpkin pudding she could eat for breakfast. It seemed like a good idea: it was a "brown thing" and had no sugar in it. However, over a couple of months of working together on her food plan, we noticed that she was becoming more and more attached to her pudding. Breakfast was important because she could have the pudding. If she skipped it for another food, she would spend the day thinking about the pudding. I really wasn't sure why this was happening, but I suggested to Anne Marie that the pumpkin pudding seemed to be acting as a trigger food and she might want to substitute something else. She agreed and changed her breakfast.

I have seen this same sort of unexpected response in my clients to several different things on the brown list, like sunflower seeds or corn products. Your job is to pay attention and notice whether any food—be it white, brown, green, or yellow—is "hooking" you. A major part of the work you are doing with this food plan is to move away from an addictive relationship to what you eat. Each person has a different response to these foods. If the food makes you crazy, sort out what is going on. Use your food journal to figure it out. Experiment. Look at the different pieces. Try new alternatives.

> Browns are important. Without browns, my girls (ages five and eight) don't do well at all and a meal won't hold them. We often add baby oatmeal to our protein shakes. It blends in really well and we all like it that way. As for cereals, we follow the rule that it has to have less than 10 grams of sugar per serving. Both my girls know how to check the labels for protein and sugar content. They love to go to the store and hunt for a new cereal that they can try. My girls love Cheerios, Clifford Crunch, Mighty Bites, and Puffins. (All but the Cheerios they discovered themselves.) Laura loves whole wheat English muffins for her morning brown. Alex loves oatmeal. Lately, Alex often does a whole wheat tortilla. Both girls are jazzed if I make whole wheat pancakes, waffles, or crepes, and I generally add protein powder and/or cottage cheese so that it has protein and brown all in one. The more I include them in the process, the easier it is. Besides, it's a lot more fun that way.
>
> —Emily

A COMPARISON OF "BROWN THINGS"

BROWN THING	SERVING	TOTAL CARBS (GRAMS)	SUGAR (GRAMS)	FIBER (GRAMS)	IMPACT
Hummus	½ cup	24.80	0.00	6.27	.00
Refried beans	½ cup	23.30	0.00	6.00	.00
Brown rice	1 cup	44.80	3.20	3.51	-.03
Sweet potato	1 medium	27.70	1.54	3.08	-.09
Baked potato with skin	1 medium	50.90	3.64	4.85	-.09
Whole-grain bread	2 slices	25.80	3.01	3.80	-.10
Oatmeal, cooked	1 cup	25.20	1.64	3.98	-.15
Pasta (whole wheat), cooked	2 cups	74.20	10.90	12.60	-.25

BROWN THING	SERVING	TOTAL CARBS (GRAMS)	SUGAR (GRAMS)	FIBER (GRAMS)	IMPACT
Quinoa	1 cup	104.20	14.11	15.98	–.25
Garbanzo beans, cooked	½ cup	22.40	4.30	6.30	–.37
Kidney beans	½ cup	20.80	3.35	5.66	–.38
Soybeans, cooked	½ cup	8.50	4.30	5.60	–.50
Black beans, cooked	½ cup	20.40	5.42	7.48	–.55
Lentils, cooked	½ cup	19.90	7.72	9.21	–.58

Source: ESHA Food Processor. Impact score by DesMaisons

"Green Things"

"Green things" are vegetables. They are a valuable part of your food plan because they are slow carbohydrates and provide lots of vitamins and minerals as well. Try to eat lots of green things. (Actually, some of your "green" things will be orange, red, yellow, or white—as in carrots, red and yellow peppers, and radishes—but "green things" is the program's shortcut term for all vegetables.) Vegetables are complex carbohydrates that have long chains of molecules and plenty of fiber, which make them slow to digest. Try to eat vegetables with both lunch and dinner. Make salad regularly. Raw vegetables are slower to digest than cooked ones; cooking vegetables breaks down their fiber instead of letting your stomach do it.

Some people who are sugar sensitive have had little experience with vegetables. If this is true for you, pick the vegetables that seem the most familiar and start with those. If preparing fresh vegetables makes you nervous, start with frozen ones. Frozen veggies are quick to make, tasty, and a simple way to get started.

Here is a list of the vegetables I eat:

Asparagus	Zucchini
Tomatoes	Cabbage
Cucumbers	Corn
Onions	Lima beans
Avocados	Parsnips
Cabbage (white and red)	Chili peppers
Eggplant	Cauliflower
Lettuce	Celery
Green beans and wax beans	Okra
Carrots	Peas
Green, red, and yellow peppers	Mushrooms
Chinese cabbage	Garlic
	Beets
	Kale

Spinach   Jicama
Broccoli   Bean sprouts
Radishes   Brussels sprouts
Squash

The next chart shows you the relative amount of fiber in some of these vegetables. The higher the ratio of fiber to total carbohydrate, the slower the carbohydrate is digested. Take a look at the listing on page 173 for Brussels sprouts. Do you see that almost half of the carbohydrate in Brussels spouts is fiber? That makes them a very slow green thing. And that's exactly why green and brown things are a better option for you than white things. It's also why we never get high from broccoli and its cousins. Have you ever heard of anyone who would kill for Brussels sprouts? For pasta maybe, but not for Brussels sprouts!

More About Fruit

Now that you have a bigger picture of carbohydrates, let's go back to the fruit story. Earlier in this chapter we saw that fruits have a fair amount of sugar. But, like brown things and green things, the impact of the sugar in fruits is tempered by the fiber they contain. The amount of fiber in the fruit affects where the fruit falls on the carbohydrate continuum. For example, raisins would fall near the left end as very, very sweet, while raspberries might fall more to the right, closer to that of broccoli. These differences make it difficult to include fruit in the carbohydrate continuum.

A separate continuum on page 174 shows only fruits so you can see how they compare with each other in terms of sugar and fiber. I generally spend a lot of time talking about fruits with my clients. Fruits become an important part of your recovery as you start to take overt sugars out of your diet. It is far too easy to slip into substituting a lot of fruit for the sugars you are trying to remove. Learn the differences in the fruit values so you don't fall into that trap.

A COMPARISON OF "GREEN THINGS"

GREEN THING	SERVING	CARBS (GRAMS)	SUGARS (GRAMS)	FIBER (GRAMS)	IMPACT
Carrots (7.5")	1	7.27	4.75	2.16	1.69
Tomato	1 medium	5.71	3.44	1.35	1.26
Pepper, green bell	1 medium	4.76	1.85	1.33	.20
Lettuce, iceberg	1 cup	1.15	0.88	.77	.08
Green peas	1 cup	22.88	8.80	8.80	0.00
Asparagus spears	6	3.81	1.44	1.44	0.00
Spinach (cooked)	1 cup	10.15	0.00	6.84	0.00
Lettuce, loose-leaf	1 cup	1.96	.90	1.06	-.08

GREEN THING	SERVING	CARBS (GRAMS)	SUGARS (GRAMS)	FIBER (GRAMS)	IMPACT
Corn	1 cup	32.14	2.95	4.43	−0.14
Green beans	1 cup	8.71	3.51	4.05	−0.22
Cabbage	1 cup	6.69	2.51	3.45	−0.35
Brussels sprouts	1 cup	12.90	5.32	6.36	−0.43
Avocado	¹/₂	7.43	.90	5.03	−0.50
Veggies, mixed, frozen	1 cup	23.84	5.82	8.01	−0.53
Broccoli	1 cup	9.84	3.31	5.52	−0.74
Lima beans	1 cup	35.10	5.04	10.60	−0.83

Source: ESHA Food Processor. Impact score by DesMaisons

THE FRUIT CONTINUUM

MOST IMPACT		MODERATE IMPACT		LEAST IMPACT	
50	40	30	20	10	0
Raisins (58)	Applesauce, sweetened (42)	Orange juice (36)	Dried figs (20)	Cherries (11)	Peach (5)
Grape juice (55)	Apple juice (39)	Prune juice (34)	Dried apricots (19)	Orange (10)	Blueberries (5)
Cranberry juice cocktail (53)		Grapes (25)	Applesauce, unsweetened (18)	Cantaloupe (10)	Plums (4)
Pineapple juice (50)			Apple, large (15)	Watermelon (9)	Strawberries (2)
			Banana (15)		Apricot, fresh (2)
			Pineapple (14)		Raspberries (1)

Serving Sizes: raisins (3 oz.); grape juice (12 fl. oz.); cranberry juice cocktail (12 fl. oz.); pineapple juice (12 fl. oz.); applesauce, sweetened (1 cup); apple juice (12 fl. oz.); orange juice (12 fl. oz.); prune juice (12 fl. oz.); grapes (1 cup); dried figs (4); dried apricots (1/2 cup); applesauce, unsweetened (1 cup); apple (large); banana (medium); pineapple (fresh, 1 cup); cherries (15); orange (large); cantaloupe (1 cup); watermelon (1 cup); peach (medium); blueberries (1/2 cup); plum (medium); strawberries (1/2 cup); apricot (1); raspberries (1/2 cup)

Look back at your food journal to see if you can discern what effect fruit has on you. Which fruits are you most drawn to? Do you like raspberries or raisins more? Look at the fiber for each. Raspberries have a lot of fiber, so the sugar hit is minimal. Raisins, on the other hand, have no fiber, and their carbohydrate is almost entirely sugar. This is why sugar-sensitive people usually prefer raisins to raspberries.

Remember what happens when you turn a whole fruit into a juice. The fiber ratio goes down because there is less fiber to slow the sugar down. The same thing happens when you cook the fruit. Look at the difference between applesauce and apples.

Also consider the impact of drying fruit. Drying fruit removes the water and makes the sugar far denser. A half cup of raisins has 63 grams of sugar, while a Coke has "only" 38, a candy bar "only" 40. You might easily snack on six pieces of dried banana even though you would never eat three whole bananas at one time. Don't be misled by the "small" portions of dried fruit. Think of them as concentrated sugar!

SHIFTING YOUR PLACE ON THE CONTINUUM

As you work with these charts, you can begin to get a sense of where you are on the carbohydrate continuum. Work at moving your eating from the left simple-carbohydrate side to the right more complex side. Experiment with your food plan to introduce little changes that support the shift. Be gentle and patient with yourself. Factor in the emotional attachment you may have to sugars or white things. Take things as slowly as you are comfortable with. And really praise yourself for whatever steps you are making in moving to the green side of the carbohydrate continuum.

THE SIXTH STEP: DEALING WITH SUGARS

In doing the first five steps, you have created a solid foundation for your recovery from the problems caused by sugar sensitivity. You have been working hard to eat in a stable and consistent way. You have started to shift your place on the carbohydrate continuum toward eating more whole grains and less white flour and sugar. You are still keeping your food journal. These tools have served you well and will continue to do so. Let's check in with where we are in the program.

THE SEVEN STEPS

1. Eat breakfast with protein.

2. Journal what and when you eat and how you feel.

3. Eat three meals a day with protein.

4. Take the recommended vitamins and have a potato before bed.

5. Shift from "white foods" to "brown foods."

6. Reduce or eliminate sugars.

7. Come alive.

Now you are ready to begin directly addressing the foods that create problems for you. Thanks to the healing you have achieved in Steps 1 to 5, you will be ready to let go of the foods that have caused so much trouble.

REDUCING OR ELIMINATING SUGARS

In Step 6, you will continue to create biochemical stability with each food and lifestyle change and begin to do the more difficult transitions. This will ensure that your food plan is safe, effective, and long-term. As you do Step 6, reducing or eliminating sugars, you will understand why I have been so insistent about taking only one step at a time. Had you tried to go off sugars your first week, you would have felt terrible. But when Step 6 is begun in the context of having successfully achieved the first five steps, your recovery from the compulsive use of alcohol, sugars, and foods made with refined white flour can be a progressive and successful process.

There is a lot of behavioral healing embedded in Step 6. The first, of course, is dealing with addiction. When you are ready to give up your "drug," you come face to face with your relationship to your "drug"—your attachment to it. Many people have no idea how powerful this is until they go to give it up.

Another piece of Step 6 is learning how to *wait*. As I am sure you know, many people come crashing in and start the program thinking that giving up sugar *now* is key. A very large part of Step 6 consists of planning, waiting, reflecting, and then taking action steps in a thoughtful way. This is huge for addicts.

A third aspect of healing embedded in Step 6 is learning what charge the different sugars carry for you. Until you are ready to give them up, it is easy to lump them all in the same pot. But straight sugar, sugar and wheat together, sugar and fat, or sugar and caffeine may all have a different charge for you. Your journal skills will have taught you this. As you do Step 6, you can tease these combinations apart and see what happens. Try caffeine without sugar and see if the charge for you is on the caffeine or the drug effect of the sugar.

When I first wrote *Potatoes Not Prozac*, I thought that Step 6 was about giving up the drug. You did that and then you were ready to roll. Through an ongoing dialogue with our community members, I began to understand that Step 6 is not an event, but a process. The process starts with achieving the stability of the first five steps, then leads into a reflection on the role of your "drug" in your life, and then into planning the best way to approach getting it out of your life. After that comes the actual "event" of reducing or eliminating sugars, followed by a fairly long time making sense of life without them. This is the process of detox, and this chapter will help you understand it and live it.

> This is outstanding! I think one of the best parts about healing is that we start to get excited about the routines of everyday life. I get a special kick out of simply watching my cats eat their breakfast every morning. I had laundry to fold this morning too, and instead of it seeming like a looming chore I actually folded and stacked with great enthusiasm. I think this is the difference—we are grateful for the daily minutiae of our lives, for the new ease we find in living. Lately I have been feeling very grateful for being sugar sensitive. After many years of suffering and I feel like I have come into the promised land.
>
> —*Karen M.*

ON THE TRAIL OF SECRET SUGARS

The discussion of the carbohydrate continuum in Step 5 gave you a good grasp of overt sugars. Now let's focus on the covert sugars.

Go back to your food journal. Using a different-colored marker, identify all the kinds of sugar you eat. Start with the overt sugars, and then mark all the other foods in which you think sugar is found. In how many places do you find sugars? Low-fat products often hide the most sugar. (When food manufacturers take out the fat, guess what they use to amp up the taste factor?)

Also take a very close look at foods that proclaim "no sugar." Remember that "no sugar" simply means "no sucrose." Manufacturers use different kinds of sweeteners to mask how much sugar is in products marketed as "healthy" or "low-fat." The labels on these foods may show five different ingredients, such as maltodextrin, raisin juice, or fructose. These all sound healthy, don't they? They are *all* sugars. Your taste buds and body will recognize them as sugars even though the label may say "sugar free." Read labels carefully. The labeling requirements demand that the manufacturer show both the "carbohydrate " and the "sugar" content. However, how the manufacturer defines "sugar" may differ from what we would call a sugar. For example, "brown rice syrup" can legally be called a "carbohydrate" because it is made from rice, which is a starch, not a sugar.

So you will have to use your brains in this process. One energy bar sold at the gym for body building has *twelve* different kinds of sugars. Of course, eating one of these would make you feel wonderful in the short run because it would spike your blood sugar level and give you a beta-endorphin hit. But you now realize that what at first feels like a positive effect is hardly that for you. This kind of energy bar will not affect your serotonin level the way a candy bar might. Can you figure out why? The energy bars also have protein in them. If you have something sweet combined with the protein you will not get a rise in tryptophan because the new aminos in the protein will still compete with little runt tryptophan. Eating sweets and protein together will not give you the serotonin effect.

Eating protein at the same time you have something sweet *will* slow down the effect on your blood sugar level. When you eat more slower, complex foods with simple ones, the digestion of the simple ones takes longer. This is why having alcohol with a meal creates less of an effect than having it without food.

Ron was doing serious body building, but he couldn't understand why his training program wasn't giving him the results he wanted. He drank gallons of Gatorade at the gym. He used "weight gain" muscle powder daily. He sincerely believed he was eating a very healthy diet. Ron had recently decided to "balance" his nutrition program and added a new meal-replacement bar. He thought he was doing everything right, but his weight and muscle development wouldn't budge. I had him bring in the ingredient labels from the meal-replacement bars and the muscle powder. We read them together and wrote down the names of the sugars they contained. It turned out that there were *nineteen* different forms of sugar in these two products. "Balanced" or not, these products didn't work for Ron. He was sugar sensitive.

Ron changed his nutrition plan to include more real food instead of the body-building supplements. He started eating three meals a day, increased his food protein, replaced "white things" with whole-grain products, and took most of the sugars out of his diet. His energy increased immediately and his endurance escalated. Within three weeks he began seeing the results in his muscle development and workout plan. What Ron had unsuccessfully worked so hard for during the past year finally started happening.

You can start learning about covert sugars the way Ron did. Read the label before you eat a food. Look at grams of sugar. It may help to visually translate grams into "teaspoons." Four grams of sugar equals one teaspoon of sugar. If a 12-ounce can of soda has 39 grams of sugar, that means you are drinking nearly 10 teaspoons of sugar with each can. If you put 10 teaspoons of sugar on a plate and look at how much it is, you may find it easier to cut down on soda!

Haha . . . I remember soon after detox, a particular time of folding laundry . . . I was so joyful about the activity itself that I felt like I must be on some sort of drug; I was simply glowing. I have been taking care of myself for a long time, but usually doing house chores for me is an obligation and I used to need A LOT of loud music playing in the background to distract myself through it. This one was quiet and every second of it felt like being in love! I was glad my mother did not see her son enjoying it so much. She is too traditional; she would be worried ;)

—*Mehmet*

The infamous "nutrition" bar says "no high fructose corn syrup," and "low fat" on the label. The ingredients (sugars and carbs are shown in italics) include: "rolled oats, *brown rice syrup* and/or Fruit Source (whole *rice syrup* and *grape juice concentrate*), rice flour, oat bran, *pear juice concentrate*, corn meal, *figs, barley malt,* cocoa powder, rice crisp, *chocolate chips,* coffee beans, natural flavors, and leavening. The label says it has 52 grams of carbohydrate, 2 grams of fiber, and 16 grams of sugars. It isn't quite clear which are the sugars and which are the carbs. But the brown rice syrup, figs, and barley malt may be classed as carbohydrates rather than sugar, even though your body will respond to them as sugars.

Because the ingredients are listed in the order of the amounts of each ingredient (this is true of *all* ingredient lists on packaged foods), the manufacturer keeps you from easily seeing that the bar is mainly sugar and oats by using seven different sugars and carbohydrates. But the large print on the label is designed to convince you what a healthy alternative this is.

Take It Easy

You may be overwhelmed when you see all the places sugars are hidden. Manufacturers like to add sugar. It makes things taste "better" and then more people will buy the product. After you have looked at a number of labels, you may wonder what you will be able to eat if you decide to eliminate sugars. Or you may have a powerful emotional response that life without sugar just isn't worth the effort. Don't scare yourself. You are just learning to read labels. Be gentle with yourself. You aren't going to take out every single sugar from your diet. You will develop good detective skills so you know where sugar lurks. This awareness will let you move from an unconscious attachment to sweets toward a conscious choice about what you eat. If you know that a can of soda has ten teaspoons of sugar, you can choose to have it or not. Conscious awareness will give you the opportunity to measure the impact. You can choose your trade-offs. You may find that it is not such a big deal to have 3 ounces of orange juice in sparkling water rather than soda because it makes you feel so much better. You may find that more and more you *like* reducing the amount of sugars you eat.

Doing Step 6 asks that you shift the way you think about what you eat. If you have been diligently keeping to a low-fat regime, you may feel cheated to have to give up sugar, too. So as you take out the sugar in your diet, you will probably increase the fat a little. But just as you shouldn't substitute sugar for fat, do not substitute fat for sugar. The name of the game is paying attention, knowing what you are eating, and noticing the effect it has on your moods and your body.

THE NEXT STEP

After you have worked at shifting to the more complex side of the carbohydrate continuum, and you have been reducing your sugars, you may decide that you are ready to go ahead and eliminate overt sugars altogether. If you feel you are ready to do this, start by thinking of the process as a detox process. You will be giving up your "drug" and will want to plan a way to minimize your discomfort and maximize your success. Thinking of going off of sugar as "detox" will also help you see that there will be predictable physiological stages and—most important—light at the end of the tunnel. Going off sugars doesn't have to be too difficult from a physical standpoint. It may be more difficult from an emotional standpoint. But we will talk about this as we go.

There is a *huge* payoff if you choose to eliminate most sugars from your diet. You will feel better than you ever have. You will still get the "good" feelings sugar has given you—the increase in serotonin and beta-endorphin—but you will get these in a new way. The skills you have developed as a food chemist and meal planner will work in your service. You will intentionally create your own good feelings with your food choices. And you will like this new state a lot.

> I treasure my sweet little morning and evening routines too. I wake up easily and naturally, let the kitties wheedle me a little with their purrs and tails, then get up and feed everybody, read RR posts, and do my morning "chores" which I feel so grateful about doing in my own dear home. It is always the same core I wake up with now. And I never go too far from it—there were times before RR when I felt adrift on an island. Now there is always music in my heart, even when I feel sad.
>
> —JoEllen

In getting ready for sugar detox, you will want look at your alcohol use. Since alcoholic beverages are the quickest sugars, they will be included in your sugar detox plan. But if you are bio-chemically dependent upon alcohol, you will experience alcohol withdrawal when you stop drinking. I want you to stay safe in the process.

Since you may not know if you have a problem with alcohol, let's take a look at a quick assessment tool to help you sort this out. Answer these four questions:

1. Have you ever felt you should cut down on your drinking?
2. Have people ever annoyed you by criticizing your drinking?
3. Have you ever felt bad or guilty about your drinking?

4. Have you ever had a drink first thing in the morning (an "eye-opener") to steady your nerves or get rid of a hangover?

If you answered "yes" to any of these questions, you may have a problem with alcohol. Plan on getting information from an alcohol specialist about the best way to address this, or come to my website at www.radiantrecovery.com for more information. See also the appendix (page 221), which is on alcoholism.

It's really helped me to participate in the lists rather than just lurk, so a big well done for coming out of the shadows and standing in where you are, however yucky that might be right now.

I got sober through the support of people on this list, and if you let us, we can be another whole arm of support in your recovery. AA has been brilliant for me, but here I find a different kind of support and adding the food element in is so important. But when my food is on track, my recovery and life just seems to be more straightforward and I'm better able to handle the challenges they both present me at times.

What I did suffer from was trying to do too much, too soon. I wanted alcohol recovery, and food recovery, and a regular gym routine, and to lose weight. And ideally, I wanted marriage and a baby too! And I want them now! Or at least within three months, thank you very much!

I've learned that we sometimes go more quickly if we strip back and go easier on ourselves. I love the phrase in AA: Keep it simple.

—H

Going Off Sugars

If you do not have a problem with alcohol (or if you had a problem in the past and are now in recovery), and you are ready to go off other sugars, go back to your food journal. This old friend will serve as your guide once again. Highlight the overt sugars you have been eating. Get a sense of what things you want to exclude from your diet. Decide whether you are going to first cut down and then cut out, or go "cold turkey." *Neither way is better.* What counts most is your style, how you like to make change in your life. Draw from the experience you have had over the past weeks and months in getting to know your own style. Do you take a gradual approach or do you plunge right in? Whichever way fits for you, use it when you create your food plan around reducing or eliminating sugars.

Most of my clients have found it easiest to first cut down as part of shifting their place on the carbohydrate continuum, then pick a time to simply go "cold turkey" and eliminate the remaining sugars in their diets. You should choose what works for you.

Planning Your Sugar Detox

Withdrawal from sugar will feel like withdrawal from a drug. This is because both sugar and narcotics raise our beta-endorphin level and when we stop using them, the brain starts begging for more. Remember, as we saw in chapter 5, sugar evokes a beta-endorphin response the same way an opiate drug like morphine or heroin does. Your withdrawal symptoms will certainly not be as severe as those of a heroin addict, but you too are physiologically going through detox. You may get the shakes, feel nauseous and edgy, or have diarrhea or headaches for a few days. You may be surprised by the intensity of the physical changes you feel. Of course, if you have tapered down the amount you are using before you do the detox, the withdrawal will not be so bad.

If you do not have any physical symptoms when you go off sugar, there are several possibilities: you didn't use a lot of sugars to begin with, you are not sugar sensitive after all, or you are getting enough covert sugar that your brain doesn't notice any change.

The sugar detox is the spectacular, visible one, but the earlier steps all are important preparation for that one. It's like looking at a curved marble staircase and forgetting to appreciate the (vital) contribution made by the wood that supports it, the form used to pour the underlying cement, the right mix of cement ingredients, the reinforcing rods of steel, and so on. The spectacular marble stairs and being free of sugar are the visible and outward effects of a lot of careful, methodical, behind-the-scenes preparation.

—*Kath*

Plan your sugar detox for a time when you do not have severe stress. The process usually takes five days, with the fourth day being the hardest. Think through the timing of your detox. Schedule it so that on the fourth day you have time to yourself. Do not start your detox so that the fourth day lands on the day you have to make a presentation to your major account. Do not plan the fourth day to coincide with your son's wedding. Be strategic.

Tell people ahead of time that because you are going off sugar, you will be going through a detox period. Get their support. If your coworker has a huge bowl of M&M's on her desk, ask her if she might put them away while you go off sugar. Plan to stay away from the places that will trigger you. Don't go into the local coffee shop even for "just coffee" until you are well through your detox. The sight or smell of the sweet rolls may trigger your cravings. I have been off sugar for many years, but I still cannot go into a Dunkin' Donuts without vividly recalling the old days when I always had two chocolate doughnuts with my coffee. The drug literature teaches us about something called "kindling," where a particular sight or smell or the memory of a certain place can activate a cascade of biochemical reactions that set off cravings.

Plan to keep your other food intake as steady as possible, and don't forget to use your food journal. This is a big step for you. If you lay the groundwork, going off sugar will not be as difficult as you might imagine, and you will feel *fabulous* when you are done.

Doing It

Your withdrawal symptoms will be minimized and you will have very few cravings if you pay special attention to your food during your detox from sugar. Drink lots and lots of water. Fill a liter bottle with water and carry it with you. Try to have two whole bottles each day. Eat more of the soluble-fiber foods like oatmeal and lentil soup because they will help to keep your blood sugar steady and minimize your cravings.

During this time, be careful about increasing the amount of fruit you are having. As you know, fruits contain sugar, and you are trying to decrease your sugar intake. If you are going to continue eating fruit, don't eat more than two pieces a day. And don't have fruit juice during your detox period.

Plan which foods you will eat for each of the five days of your detox. You may feel crabby and irritable during this period and not want to go to the grocery store or have to plan meals. Prepare for this time so you will feel supported and optimistic that you can do it.

Your full sugar detox takes about five days. On the first day you'll feel excited about getting started. On day two you may begin to feel irritable and edgy. On days three and four, you may be physically uncomfortable with a headache, joint pain, or upset stomach. You get these symptoms because you have beta-endorphin receptor sites in these places, too. When these sites don't get the "drug" they are used to, they let you know—with symptoms. You may feel irritable, angry, tense, or jittery. You may have difficulty concentrating or remembering things. You may wonder why you ever started this detox in the first place.

Day four, the hardest day, will be crucial. If you get really uncomfortable, have a piece of fruit. No, don't eat four bananas. One will do. Or have an apple or some strawberries. Don't have raisins or figs even if they call to you. Remember, you are close to being done with the actual event of detox. Hang in there. If you can manage to get through it, on day five you'll feel great! You'll have energy and will feel more stable than you can remember. Coming through a sugar detox will feel good.

Your detox may take a little longer or a little shorter depending on how much you had reduced your sugar intake before you started this phase. Obviously, if you had already taken most sweet things out over time, this phase will be pretty simple. If you decided to be dramatic and go from everything (eating lots of "white things" and sugars) to nothing, you will have a dramatic detox—you will feel terrible and then will feel wonderful. We have thousands of people who have done the drama detox. They feel fabulous and on top of the world—then they crash and burn and come back to the program somewhat chastened. In reality, you want your brain chemistry to be able to keep up with your enthusiasm, and that takes a little time.

After you have completed your sugar detox, allow yourself some time to get used to your new way of eating. Keep doing your food journal, and let yourself notice how your food plan is going. Stay steady. Keep eating lots of protein, "brown stuff," and "green stuff." Keep eating three meals a day at regular intervals. Keep taking your vitamins. And enjoy how you feel.

Alcoholics Anonymous talks about living "one day at a time." With sugar recovery, one day at a time won't work. You will need to live your recovery one choice at a time. In the first stages after detox, don't think about never having sugar again. That concept is a killer. Don't even try to consider it. Just let yourself stay focused on one choice at a time. Don't even stretch it to one day at a time. Stick with one choice at a time. At the moment you walk into the coffee shop, ask yourself whether you can choose not to have a scone with your coffee. At the moment you get in line at the grocery store on your way home from work, ask yourself if you can choose not to buy a Butterfinger to munch in the car on the way home. Don't make it any bigger than each little choice like these.

Although many of the physical feelings are similar, going off sugars differs from going off alcohol or drugs in a huge way:

You can't just put "the bottle" away. You will have to make food choices every day, many times a day. Going off sugars is a very big deal. Give yourself the recognition and credit for doing a fabulous job on something that is very difficult.

> I've been "osockrad" (unsweetened), as my friend calls it, for ten days now and I feel great! I seem to notice other things more than before. For example, I see that I need a little more protein in my lunch. Journaling is easier, too, I seem to receive more and better information. I feel a little vulnerable though, doing life without sugar, like you said without my comfort. But I'm sure that will pass.
>
> —Lisa, Sweden

The time after detox can be a little disorienting. Many of you have been drama queens or adrenaline junkies. You are used to creating chaos by leaving bills till they are overdue, not paying taxes, forgetting a key appointment, having a fight with your husband, wife, partner, or children, blowing up at work, having a temper tantrum, whatever. You get a rush from the drama. When you start the program and work the steps, you experience a plan designed to *minimize* drama. You learn to cope with thoughtful planning rather than reaction and mobilization. You create behavioral change. When you learn not to eat until mealtime in Step 3, you learn to wait and to tolerate discomfort.

At first, you will feel a sense of elation that you have actually accomplished what you set out to do. Over time, you may feel "flat" because the spiky life that comes with addiction is quiet. You will need to learn to tolerate some flatness rather than creating drama, and you may label this time as "boring."

As we started to process this feeling with people in our one Step 6 group (called a "list" in Web terminology), we discovered that everyone experienced it. This was when we decided that we needed to think of Step 6 not as an event but a process. The flatness seems to last for about six months. Then some miracle happens. The flatness becomes "the Calm." I will talk more about this in the chapter on Step 7. First I want you to hear Cinzia, who wrote a remarkable description of the Step 6 process.

The actual detox was uneventful and there I was. Then I felt volatile for several months, like I was on a pitching, rolling ship. I'd be calm for a few days, then a "rogue wave" came along and knocked me for a little loop. It wasn't spiky, but it was up and down. I usually couldn't find any explanation for it from the data in my journal. And I didn't like it!

Just knowing that other people had experienced the same thing helped me. I kept doing the food, being as consistent as I could. I tried not to worry about the ups and downs, and just kept going. I ate more browns some of the time and ate *a lot* of nuts. After the volatility came the Calm. Really, it was like the aftermath of a storm. I caught my breath and was glad for a bit of rest. Then the Calm kept going. And I realized that my body, mind, and soul needed this time to integrate some of the enormous changes that were going on. I started to appreciate Calm.

These last few weeks I feel like I'm getting my spark back. I feel more buoyant most days. It's a different quality, hard to describe. Not spiky or dramatic. Just more effervescent some of the time. I guess it's radiance, eh?

—*Cinzia*

12

THE SEVENTH STEP: COMING ALIVE

Doing Step 7 is quite different from your experience with the other steps. After your brain gets settled and you have a sense of life without your "drug," Step 7 just starts to creep in. It does not have a specific task. It is a developmental process that emerges as the initial flatness after sugar detox becomes the Calm.

So the first phase of Step 7 is the Calm, the place of ease and rest where you no longer have to live in drama. Then comes the active phase of Step 7, exploring your new life and learning new skills. You are going to learn how to have a life without your "drug." At first, this will be very exciting. Getting here is a huge accomplishment. But it can also be disorienting.

You may have felt that Step 7 was the top of the mountain, the ultimate destination. But Step 7 is really the beginning of another complete process. You no longer have the same structure to follow as in the earlier steps. It is like being a grown-up and being out in the world on your own.

Another thing I've been noticing is that I'm much more able to do one thing at a time. And there's a specificity about that one thing. Before, I would want to do 10,000 things, but they would all be vague or too big. Now, it's not "clean the house," it's "get a garbage bag and walk from room to room, collect the trash, and put it out." I have a much better sense of what I can do with a chunk of time.

—Tom

One very important tool is the connection to others who are further along in the journey. Learning the skills of life in recovery is hard. You used to turn to sweets or alcohol to take care of the complex or painful stuff. Now you may feel raw and a little disoriented. Then you get an even bigger shock. You realize that the people around you are *not* in recovery, and, *whew,* it is hard!

When you are looking at your life through the filter of recovery, you see things that you may have been in denial about. Addiction buffers you from the ugly nature of the things around you. You may have a dysfunctional marriage or family, you may have settled for a dysfunctional job. There are any number of other things you will face for the first time. When you get steady with your food, and then turn around to look at your life, it isn't all pretty.

This can be quite unsettling because *now* you see, *now* you feel. You are no longer in sugar-driven denial. So you have to learn how to wait and stay settled without getting all perturbed or needing to fix everything. You learn to focus on doing the food and trusting that the changes that you might want to make will simply become clear to you over time. The good news is, because of your recovery, you won't freak out about what you see. Still, feeling unsettled is unsettling. This is another time when having support from others in the program is very helpful.

Some people come into Step 7 thinking that all will be rosy. They are very disconcerted at how hard the early transition period is. As you talk with others, though, you will discover that you are able to work it through. It is uncomfortable but not impossible. You no longer get overwhelmed or angered. By Step 7, you have a biochemical clarity that will serve you well—as will the practice you had in the earlier steps with journaling and adjusting your choices based on what you notice. These are life skills. The more you use them, the more your program deepens.

The skill-building part of Step 7 is about tackling the things that you didn't do so well before your recovery and the things you chose not to look at. The more you tackle these now, the more your life changes. The flatness starts taking on color. Flat becomes Calm. And something in you starts to like it. Really like it. Eighteen months in and drama no longer holds the same appealing charge. You find yourself wanting to deescalate rather than amp up. Now the drama seems like a waste of energy you could use on fun things.

Before, my focus was just on the food, and I let the rest take care of itself. I couldn't see how I would ever understand all that other stuff. Yet all that "hard" stuff is becoming easier now and I think that is the change. I feel more, well, calm and able, I think. I notice more what is going on inside me, I guess that is cos I am able to do the food pretty well automatically, and so other things want my attention!

So the books say Step 7 is about getting a life . . . so I figure it's about enriching your life and building the things that keep your BEs [beta-endorphin] steady into your daily routine and also, as I get further through Step 7, I guess my "big" self will start to emerge and I will see if I'm on course for what I truly want to do with my life and be able to change it if it isn't. I think I should be able to get steady on other things like exercise and stuff on Step 7 and will be able to look at weight loss issues too.

—*Milly*

Then another change creeps in. Rather than being a drama queen or adrenaline junkie, you become funny and creative. Your innovative self starts flourishing. You are flexible and resourceful. You deal well with crisis, you are proactive in problem-solving. All sorts of things start to change. *Who is this person?* you might ask. When you started this program, you thought it was about controlling your food. Now, in Step 7, you start to understand that life without addiction is truly remarkable.

Here is a quick list of some of the things the members of our community have identified as changing over time once they are on Step 7:

- They clear up their problems with money.
- They start setting healthy boundaries.
- They look at relationships with new eyes.
- They heal shame.
- They heal old emotional wounding.
- They clear their clutter, both emotional and physical.
- They leave unsatisfying jobs.
- They go back to school.
- They start following their dreams and living their passions.

Chances are, you will experience Step 7 in the same way. You will fearlessly look at stuff as it comes up, you will get help as needed, you will take care of it, and you will move forward.

While you are in this process, you may yearn for the structure of the earlier steps. You may want the ease of knowing what will happen next. But eventually something changes. A new level of emotional maturity emerges as you step further away from your sugar addiction, and further toward your brilliant future.

The ability to work without structure is part of the growing-up process. Remember the first time in school when you had free rein? Remember when you had to write something without the aid of lined paper? Or the

difference between the pacing and verifying of high
school assignments versus the independence of college
work? That's how I see Step 7. It's moving on to a new
phase where you have a lot more latitude, and it's time
for you to have that latitude because the foundation has
been laid and you are ready for it.

—*Elaine*

After a while, Step 7 calls you to think about what you want
your life to be. Your heart starts strumming its desire for meaning.
A yearning begins to whisper in your ear about life. Jobs, relationships, healing spirituality, they all start changing.

I am floored at how consistent the changes are. People on
Step 7 share in our online community about their freedom from
the tyranny of sugar addiction, the incredible changes in their
health, and their monumental life changes—things they never
expected! Something is happening here. "Doing the food" creates change at a much deeper level than you might have ever
imagined.

This time is very interesting because I've noticed my
energy and interest shifting to the small, the practical,
the doable, the finite. In short, it's a feeling of "daily
practice." At first, there were a lot of little voices in my
head saying things like, "Where's your ambition? Don't
you want to be SOMEBODY?" You know what? Those
voices have gone away. I have other messages that keep
whispering to me, "Live each day." "Slow down and love
today." "Love the people around you." "Stop hurrying."
"Enjoy the abundance you already have." My life feels
like it's slowed down to a manageable pace, and it's more
fun—a lot more fun!

Before, each day was a checklist of things to get done
to further my nebulous ambition. Now when someone
talks to me, I'm actually there and listening to them. I

don't have to hold everything in my head. One thing is
starting to flow into the next, and I feel calm about that.
I don't need to have a Master Plan anymore. Obviously, I
have the structure of the steps, but they are infrastructure
now—quietly whirring away. It's not "Omigod, all I think
about is: Have I done the steps today?"

—Vinny

When your food is consistent, regular, and on target, there
is just no more drama. The program gets more and more simple.
You do the food, do the laundry, talk with friends (I added that
because it was all sounding a little solitary), brush the dogs and
cats, mop the floor, go get groceries, meditate, and exercise. And
while you do, radiance breathes you into healing.

13

LIVING YOUR RADIANT RECOVERY

Now it is time to start thinking about the long haul. Over time, you may come to feel that this program is too simple. The idea of eating breakfast may seem silly. Because I am not giving you sheets and sheets of instructions to follow, you may decide this plan isn't really right for you. You may start, do your food journal for a week, get bored with it, and decide to go off sugar all at once. A week later you are scarfing up really "healthy" energy bars since you know these will give you energy. Of course you feel a whole lot better in the short run. You think you have given up sugar and can lose weight now by eating only two "meals"—an energy bar for breakfast, no lunch, and a "healthy" dinner of pasta and salad. Everything seems fine. This plan wasn't for you after all.

A few months down the road, you notice that you are having three double lattes each day with a bran muffin in the morning, an energy bar as a midmorning snack (and another later before your workout), pasta salad for lunch, and brown rice with vegetables for dinner. You have added two glasses of wine before dinner. Or you may have simply slipped back to having two double lattes in the morning on the way to work. Breakfast isn't really that important. And you know that eating will make you fat.

Your energy keeps slipping away, especially in the late afternoon, so you add some more caffeine then to help finish the day. You aren't sleeping too well, but you make no connection to the food you are eating, and you assume your fatigue is from job stress. You start getting irritable at work. There's too much to do, not enough time. Your boss is getting on your nerves. You need to stop off for a drink before going home. Weekends bring low-fat whole-grain pancakes instead of the muffin, but much of your days off are spent trying to catch up with your life.

What is wrong with this picture? Your food is low-fat, "healthy." You ask yourself, "Why am I feeling terrible here? Maybe I need to exercise more." You take a "carbohydrate and electrolyte replacement" drink with you to the gym. (These drinks are water with sugar and salt.) Your energy goes up before the workout, you feel better. Exercise must be the key. But a few weeks later, it's not working. What is the matter here? You can hardly get out of bed. You feel like a truck ran over you.

The answer is simple. Your body is sensitive to sugar. Your blood sugar is spiking and crashing all day. You have huge beta-endorphin releases all day (which are causing downregulation and triggering cravings), and you don't have enough protein, so you aren't getting the tryptophan your body needs to make the serotonin you need to do your life. A traditional food plan or diet will not provide the answer to your problem.

My solution is simple, but it takes commitment. Eating breakfast or writing down your food every day requires commitment. You can easily dismiss or forget these steps. "I forgot my book." "I went on a trip." "I got busy." "I got bored." Thousands of reasons subvert the process. But your body will remember what it felt like when you ate the way it needs you to. You will have a molecular memory of what I call "radiance." You can always go back to that place.

The more you can approach this process with humor and appreciation for the long haul, the more you can hang in there with it over time. Most diet plans work for only a little time. Then the book sits on your shelf, reminding you of yet one more program that sounded good but didn't work for you. This time you are learning skills rather than following sheets and sheets of instructions.

Remember, twelve-step programs advise taking life "one day at a time." But when you are in a crisis with your food and you don't feel good, a day is way too long. Take your life *one choice at a time*. Only one choice. This commitment is all you have to make. Start with breakfast. Make the choice to eat real food for breakfast. Make the choice to have protein. Go back to your food journal. Pay attention to what's happening for you. Find someone to support your process.

ACTIVITIES TO SUPPORT YOUR RADIANT RECOVERY

All through this book you have heard me talk about finding support. I continue to stress this because I know that sugar-sensitive people with their low levels of beta-endorphin have a natural inclination to try to "tough it out." When we are very little, we experience the emotional sense of isolation that comes with low beta-endorphin. So we adapt. We learn to get by on our own. We don't operate from an inherent sense of connectedness to others, and we don't realize that this pattern has shaped our way of being in the world. It just seems as if we are busy or shy and we simply don't move well in circles of shared experience.

You have already started moving out of this lifelong pattern by making the biochemical changes that come with changing your food. You may find that now you are open to the idea of support but haven't a clue how to start. And your usual sources of support might not be the best place.

Your family may have a mixed response to your doing this food plan. Initially, they may feel skeptical about you going on "one more diet." When you get to the sugar detox, they may feel horrified that you are going to take away their sugars, too. But as you make changes in the way you eat, you will become more settled,

more relaxed, and more energetic. Your family will notice this—
the death of Dr. Jekyll/Mr. Hyde will not pass unnoticed—and
they are going to want to know what is going on. Share George's®
Shake with them. Share the alternatives to simple carbohydrates
that you have discovered. You may find they get excited and want
to do the food plan with you. (Do be careful that in their excite-
ment they don't co-opt your food so you are left without the sup-
plies you need for your own plan.)

Or they may decide that they do not want to have anything
to do with this plan. They may be incredibly resistant or totally
uninterested in anything that has to do with eating more regularly
and giving up sugar. They may even actively subvert your commitment to the plan. Your husband may ask, "Aren't you done
with that experiment yet?" as he orders a bottle of your favorite
wine or takes a big forkful of a dessert that you would kill for. Your
wife may say, "Aren't you going overboard?" Your partner may say,
"You don't expect me to do this with you, do you?" Your kids may
come rushing home with "Mom, look what I brought you!" And
they hand you the cookies they know you shouldn't eat, hoping
they can eat them instead. Remember, sugar sensitivity is inherited. Your children may be cookie lovers too.

Your friends may not be the best support option either. A close
friend who is still very attached to chocolate or French bread may
warn you of the dangers of a "high-protein diet." Telling him or
her that this food plan is not a high-protein diet will have no
impact because the issue isn't really about protein at all. The issue
is about their resistance to your change. If you change, they may
have to. And people in resistance are not ready for change. This
is why you need support from people who understand your process
and your program. Talking with other folks who are supportive is
absolutely critical to your success.

Dr. Kathleen saved my life. I crawled out of the depths of
darkness and despair and am more "even" every day. The

sun is brighter, the grass is greener, my vision is clear now. No more hangovers. I love life and face the challenges with a no-problems-just-solutions attitude. I know that this program is vital to my well-being, and I trust it completely. My journal is the first thing I reach for in the morning (along with a big glass of water). Then I sit and read all of your posts. You are my morning hugs, grateful list, and friends. You are wonderful and awesome.

—*Kathy*

You simply need to connect with other sugar-sensitive people who are doing the program. The combination of a healing message and fellowship is a powerful duo. When I first published *Potatoes Not Prozac* in 1998, I wanted to create a healing community for sugar-sensitive people around the world. I knew that the Internet could do this. So I designed a website to foster community: www.radiantrecovery.com. There is no charge to be a part of this magnificent group. Go see.

Gee, I have been in tears most of the time reading the posts! I had the same thing last week, when I discovered the forum. Not ready to answer yet, I read and read and cried and cried, feeling like coming home. . . . It is all so warm and friendly, and many of the posts are so "my story"! I feel welcomed and embraced into a family I have missed for such a long time. I feel more "normal," and not as "weird" as I have always felt (about my food). Thank you all so very much!!

(O, and the practical stuff is very clear too, I have checked out the steps and they work well.)

—*Tessa, Netherlands*

People reading my books found the Radiant Recovery® site, and started talking with each other via online chats. I listened and offered guidance. I added specialized "lists" in response to the needs I heard. I read every single email and post that was sent to the site. As the community grew, I identified those people doing the program who were natural leaders, and I trained and nurtured them to work with other sugar-sensitive people coming to the site. I insisted that the leadership team live the program and not just talk about doing it.

Today the Radiant Recovery® website has more than 500 pages, 140 specialized lists with more than 250,000 posts on them, a forum that has 250,000 posts, several weekly chats, and a community that represents more than 80 countries.

> I just love chat. I don't think I've missed one Eurochat yet. I am so grateful we have our own chat, too. It has really made my program come together. Attending chat makes me feel normal when I feel burdened by my sugar sensitivity. It makes me feel part of something. I always log off feeling cheered, enthused, encouraged, inspired, and intrigued. It's the best!
>
> —Milly, London

Here are some of the specific resources you will find. We have a series of orientation classes that will show you how the site works, what is in the resource center, and what is in the Radiant Recovery® store. We have a support group/list for every step. There is no charge for any of the support groups/lists. We have inexpensive online classes about brain chemistry, each of the seven steps, and special topics like depression, IBD, anxiety, and sleep. We have a special support network for people dealing with alcohol. Parents talk with one another and learn to use my book *Little Sugar Addicts* to help their children and their families make changes. We have a separate online program for people wanting to lose weight using the concepts outlined in my fourth book, *Your Last Diet!*

We also have groups/lists for fun, like gardening and pets, and we have added a number of hospitality groups/lists that enable people who live near each other to make face-to-face connections. These are organized by region in the United States and include groups in Canada, the United Kingdom, Scandinavia, and Australia. As more people join the community and want to connect with each other, we expand the hospitality groups to welcome them. We also have regional seminars and hold an annual retreat (I call it "the ranch") both in Albuquerque, where I am based, and in the United Kingdom.

> I find it magic that I can be in South Africa sharing with other sugar sensitive people from all around the world. This is technology at its best.
>
> —Karen, South Africa

Despite this phenomenal growth in the size of our community, each person coming in is led through a simple orientation, given a personal welcome, and shown how to find just what she or he needs. Radiant Recovery® works as a community because it is led by people who want to give back by "giving forward" for the healing they have received. As their own recovery grows, they are more and more able to serve as trusted guides in the process for the new people coming in.

> I subscribed to your newsletter to keep myself on track. I have already gone through your program and detoxed in January 2003. I lost 86 pounds altogether and have kept it off. I am forty-eight years old and I am the fittest I have ever been and feel great. I started your program in October 2001 and took each step slowly and didn't move on till I felt comfortable. It took me fifteen months to get to Step 6 but well worth it. I got a lot of support from your website and the community forum. I am very

grateful for that. Many events have happened since my
detox including my husband leaving me and getting a
divorce but I didn't let those events distract me from my
goal. I am very grateful for your books and this program.
I am truly radiant.

—Caroline

The combination of this book and the Radiant Recovery®
community means that your process can go way beyond simply
reading these pages and feeling that the information is useful.
It means that you have a wealth of tools you need to transform
your life.

SAFEGUARDING YOUR PROGRESS

The road to radiance can take many paths. Here is a diagram that shows three of the more typical routes that people take. The paths and the stories are composites of thousands of real people. Imagine each of these shows a three-year period.

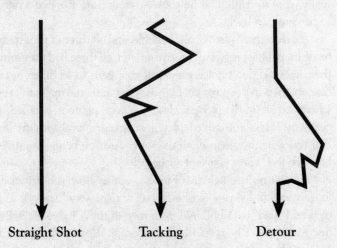

Straight Shot   **Tacking**   **Detour**

The first, the one I call the straight shot, is the path of someone who had ten years in Alcoholics Anonymous when she started my program. She had a lot of life skills, but she simply did not feel well. She was depressed. Life seemed to be leaving her behind. She read the first edition of *Potatoes Not Prozac* and recognized her story. She did the steps slowly and in order, and she focused on the food. She connected with the Radiant Recovery® online community, she joined the support groups, she took classes, and she did not fret. Her program simply got better and better. Of course, we might add a disclaimer to this one as "results not typical."

The second route is that of a woman who did a lot of what I call tacking. She was young, she was sure she knew how to do the program better than the rest of us. She believed she was a special case, so she tried a lot of things along the way. But she really wanted recovery, she really wanted radiance, so she always came back to the steps and got settled again after her wandering. She made progress over time, even though at any given point she might have been off trying some new diet.

The third path belongs to a guy who loved the program from the start. He moved right along. Then he decided that beer was really okay for him, and he took a detour. Life stopped working, so he came on back.

All three paths are equally possible, and all three of these people made incredible progress. Three years later, all three had transformed their lives. So don't judge yourself if your path looks different from that of others in the program. Let *your* program settle in. Think about where you are in the process. Have you been rigorous, detailed, and persistent? Have you dallied, played, or poked around with the steps? Are you weighing yourself all the time? Are you being attentive to how you feel? Have you kept a journal?

As you go through this process, notice how you criticize or judge yourself. Do you ascribe "good" to rigorous adherence to the plan and "bad" to dabbling? Listen to your inner judge carefully to discover if she or he is an ally or a saboteur. Work with those inner voices. They are crucial to your long-term success. This process may not work the way you might expect. For example, sometimes diligence is less useful than dalliance. For many, many years you told yourself to be self-disciplined. You have pushed yourself and felt guilty when you couldn't do what you demanded of yourself. Perhaps there is a different way of doing things. Perhaps we can change your relationship to your body *and* your relationship to yourself.

> I thought I would check in for a little. Things are going really well for me. I'm getting ready to start back up for the year with the lawn biz. I can't wait to get started; I'm really excited about it this year. It is so nice to be able to work for myself and do something that I love doing.
>
> Food is stable. I try to keep in mind those sayings of Kathleen's, like "if you want what we have, do what we do." If the food is wobbly, then life is wobbly, if the food is steady, then life is steady.
>
> Currently I have my sights set on one heck of a rather large trout I have found. I have named him KONG! We have had some melting and rain so the streams are up and unfishable right now, but as soon as they lower I'm going after him again. I had him hooked last week but he managed to escape the grip of the troutfisherguy lol. I know where he lives, and I will catch him again sooner or later, and once I do I will take pics of Kong, and then release him back to his domain.
>
> — *Tom*

When I first started doing my own plan, I thought that "getting" the program meant doing it fully, being diligent, following the instructions, and not messing with it. I still held the belief that being disciplined and focused were the only ways to go. Now I am not so sure that these are the criteria for succeeding with the program.

Now I am convinced that something else is operating, something a little more subtle and unexpected. I believe that showing up and being in relationship to your body will help you more than being tough on yourself. Let me outline how I got to thinking this way.

I used to lead a ten-week guided imagery series called "Finding Healing From Within." Each week we would do a guided meditation. After the meditation, the participants would draw what they experienced, and the group would share their feelings. Sometimes group members would sleep through every single meditation and make up a drawing because they had no memory of anything in the meditation. This made me really uncomfortable. Was I failing these people? Were they failing the group? Were they in denial? How could they sleep through my wonderful imagery?

At the end of ten weeks, we reviewed the progress of everyone in the group. How had they changed? How did they feel? Surprisingly, time and time again, the sleepers would have as remarkable a change as the doers. Not once, not twice, but every single time. Ten weeks of sleeping through what I thought was the healing part of the work and they would report a profound sense of inner healing. They didn't work it. They slept through the meditation—at least on a conscious level. But they were there. They showed up and they drew the pictures and they talked about their process.

This experience taught me something. The act of showing up creates change. In fact, it creates powerful change even if on the outside it may not seem so. Making a commitment to healing starts a process—a chain of events that is much deeper than we may think. When you vow, "I will get better," when you begin to hold the idea of being willing to do whatever it takes, then something starts to shift.

Given this experience with my "sleepers," I looked again at the effect that dalliance versus diligence might have on the seven steps of healing sugar sensitivity. I started looking at my personal process of doing the steps. What was happening when I was playing around with them a little instead of being diligent? Could those times be like the sleeping times in my guided imagery class? Could change be happening in spite of what seemed to be my own inattention? I looked in my food journal and discovered something astounding. When I was attending to the steps, listening to my body, writing in my journal, even if I wasn't doing the food plan perfectly, change was happening. I was making progress even when I was being kind of sloppy.

Think about those sleepers. The sleepers were there in the room with the rest of the group. Every week. They woke up, drew pictures with the group, and talked about sleeping. And when I showed up, kept my food journal, and wrote about sleeping through my food plan, I was still engaged with my body and working the steps. I was talking with myself about what was happening. I was not criticizing myself for "food sleeping." I was simply noticing. And I kept coming back to the journal. I kept coming back to my body and my healing.

The nature of the sugar-sensitive person is to give in when things get difficult. Like the C57 mice, you crouch in the corner and think you can't stick to your plan. Your biochemistry and your coping behaviors have supported learned helplessness. You hit hard stuff and you felt overwhelmed, unable to follow through the way you hoped. A thousand failed diets from the past reinforced these feelings. As soon as you catch yourself "sleeping," you say to yourself, "See, you did it again!" So you run away from the program, run away from yourself. You crouch and hide—and then you abandon everything you have learned.

This time it will be different, because knowing you are sugar sensitive lets you finally, finally understand the nature of who you are. Knowing you are sugar sensitive lets you shift the perspective from feeling bad about a thousand "failed" diets to being open to a solution. Think about that. You are tenacious. You keep going, you search and continue. You may be impulsive and impatient, but you can be and are committed to finding a solution.

This program helps you use your tenacity in a new way. Because you finally understand why other diets haven't worked, you can start to make choices. You can change the voices that say, "I know this won't really work" into "Hmmmm, let's sort this out," "Why am I bored?" "Why don't I like doing the journal?" "Why do I sabotage my efforts?" Asking these questions becomes a part of your healing. They are not the same old tapes you have run about your inadequacy. They may be the same questions, but they are asked from a different perspective.

Say to yourself, "I will do whatever it takes to heal this. I will give it time, money, energy, whatever it takes. Taking care of my food will be at the *top* of my list, not after my job, or after my family, or maybe when I get to it. But at the top of my list every day." You have made these affirmations a thousand times. But generally you make them in your head. You think about your affirmations, but you do not usually put the affirmations into action. What would it really mean to "do whatever it takes"?

All of you will have slippery times or times when you just go right off track. This is totally normal. We are more interested in progress rather than perfection. I honestly believe there is *no* failure in this program. There are simply opportunities to learn more about yourself and to keep going.

I have to share what a moving and profound experience last night's chat was for me. The whole ambivalence, commitment, fear thing is exactly what I have been working through the last few months as I struggled to figure out why I never got beyond Step 2. It happened just like Kathleen said—I got friendly with my ambivalence and I found my fear: I am afraid of where radiance might take me. I cannot imagine me radiant. But once I found the fear and could name it, I was able to commit to healing anyway. I post whether I feel like it or not. I eat three meals a day whether I feel like it or not. And this doesn't feel like self-discipline, it just feels like "doing it" because I want to heal rather than to hide in my fear. Journaling is even getting easier.

So last night I sat in front of my computer with a lump in my throat and tears in my eyes because Kathleen was putting my life into words, and I could see that I will be radiant one day and I won't be afraid anymore.

—*Janice*

Your skill set needs to include what to do when you get in trouble. As your program progresses, you will become more and more adept at catching the warning signals that your food is off. Here are some things to watch for:

- Irritability
- Fatigue
- General edginess
- Thinking that goes around and around
- Feeling on edge
- Emotional fragility
- Low tolerance for stress
- Inability to concentrate
- Feeling inadequate

These are the warning signs. Remember that trouble is not when you consciously have three pieces of chocolate cake. It's when you lapse into unconsciousness and have French bread one day, a bagel the next, a glass of wine the next, and then three pieces of chocolate cake. Trouble isn't a single event. It's the *process* of losing touch with how vulnerable you are to addiction. Trouble starts way earlier than full-blown sugar relapse. It starts with little "justas." Having "justa" slice of French bread, and "justa" bagel or glass of wine. Things creep in and you stop journaling because you do not want to see them. Then you are sliding down the slide. Your addictive brain will say, "Well, this is not a full-blown relapse. I can get back on track." But you never quite get to it. So you slip and slide for months or years.

After you get off a drug (remember that sugar *is* a drug) for a while, your neuroreceptors upregulate to compensate for the change. So if you have not had sugars for a while, your brain has opened up more beta-endorphin receptors in an attempt to capture whatever beta-endorphin they can. This makes you a sitting duck for relapse unless you pay very close attention. If you have some sugar, you are going to feel fabulous because you now have lots and lots of receptor sites to grab the beta-endorphin evoked by the sugar. So the "justa" sugar you ate will prime the beta-endorphin system, and you will start to experience huge cravings. This propels you into full-blown relapse.

Here's what it can look like:

Marcy reports that she had a major slip. She ate a huge piece of chocolate cake. Since then she has had a really hard time getting stabilized. She says she feels as if the floodgates opened and all she wants is sweet things and bread. She sincerely believes the chocolate cake did it. She goes back to her food journal and begins highlighting the sugars she had in the week prior to the chocolate cake.

She discovers that the sugar actually started creeping in about ten days earlier. She was under a lot of stress at work. Someone offered her half a bagel midmorning. She ate it and noted feeling much better, really relaxed. The next evening she went out to dinner and was really "hungry" so she snacked on French bread before the meal came. She only had "one or two" pieces and didn't think about it at all. The next day, she was "hungry" midmorning so she decided to get a cinnamon roll with her decaf coffee at 11:00 a.m.

She didn't notice what was happening. The following day, she felt edgy midmorning. She attributed it to PMS. After work, the kids really got on her nerves. Dinner was running late, they were crabby, she was climbing the walls. The kids came in and got cookies and milk for a snack since she had told them dinner would be late. She felt angry at having to fix dinner anyway. They left the cookie bag on the counter.

Marcy poured herself a glass of milk saying, "This is better than drinking wine," and then absentmindedly chomped five cookies while she prepared dinner. The next morning she got up with a headache and felt really edgy. The day was one of high stress on the job. She never got a chance to eat lunch. It was a special occasion so her husband picked her up for dinner. They went to a nice restaurant and had a very pleasant meal. Karen felt ravenous so she ate bread to start, then had pasta with fresh tomatoes and basil.

After dinner, she ordered a cappuccino, and the man with

the dessert tray walked by. There in front of her sat a piece of dark chocolate cake with raspberry sauce dribbling over the side. Since this was a special occasion, she decided that it would be okay to have the cake "just this once." Marcy and her husband had a wonderful evening. She skipped breakfast the next day, had pasta salad on the run for lunch, ate cookies after work, and by dinnertime was ready to kill.

Her appointment with me came the following day. She woke up then and told me about the "slip" with the cake at the restaurant. As I led her through the past week, Marcy began to see that the cake was really not the slip. In fact there really wasn't an "event." Instead there was creeping neurotransmitter interest in the euphoric effect of the sugars. Thousands of upregulated beta-endorphin receptors were just singing at the idea of being stimulated. "More, more!" they were shouting.

The trick to feeling your best is to create a highly balanced system. You do not want a seriously upregulated system with your receptors shouting for more. You don't want to prime the little suckers unless you know exactly what you are doing. Unconscious flirtation with sugar-induced euphoria will put you in a very vulnerable place. Your biochemistry will lead you to repeat your actions. Stimulating the beta-endorphin will activate priming. You will feel good and want to do it again. The key here is *paying attention*. Read your food journal, use your yellow highlighter. Know what is happening with your food and your life.

You goal is not to go off sugar for the rest of your life. Your goal is to become aware of what, how, and when you eat every day. Going off sugar and changing your food habits is not like going off alcohol, drugs, or nicotine. You do not have a day when everything shifts and you become totally abstinent. If you set yourself to believe that you will be totally abstinent for the rest of your life, you are simply setting yourself up for failure. Doing a food plan doesn't work that way. It is a *process* of becoming more aware, more attentive, more committed as you go. If you have a cinnamon roll, you need to stop and reflect on what is going on. Listen to your body.

Listen very closely. Learn to recognize not only behavioral clues but emotional clues and even neurological ones.

Over time, you will come to know the difference between the effects of serotonin decline, beta-endorphin priming, and a low blood sugar reaction. Each of these has distinctly different symptoms and effects in your body. Your job is to become the leader of the pack. Don't let your impulses take over. *Choose* your response, your way of dealing with what your body is asking for.

- If you find yourself feeling *impulsive and irritable*, flying off the handle, you are experiencing low serotonin. Start knitting, and be really attentive about ol' Mr. Spud at bedtime. Be in service to your healing.
- If you feel *grumpy and start drifting toward sugar things*, go for a vigorous walk to raise your beta-endorphin level.
- If you feel *muddy and unfocused* (this can be either low serotonin or low beta-endorphin), as if you're in a fog, go for a brisk walk and get your body moving.
- If you feel *fuzzy-headed and shaky*, stop and have a snack right away to raise your blood sugar.

Remember, though, that all these are clues that you need to tighten your program. Do not think in terms of a short-term "antidote," think about the steps, think about your food. Steady program means feeling good almost all the time. Living this way will give you confidence and awareness. Rather than being the victim of your inherited body chemistry, you will find joy and delight in your sensitive and complex system. Your inquiring brain will find that food becomes a fun and powerful tool for feeling better and better.

STOPPING THE JOURNAL

There will come a point when you want to stop keeping your food journal. Assess what lies behind this decision. You may be bored with having to do it—or you may not like what you see. You may be frustrated by the fact that you can't maintain your food plan. If this is the case, continue with your journal anyway, even if you aren't happy about the task.

On the other hand, you may feel you have truly mastered a food plan that works for you and feel you have gone beyond the need to do the journal. If that's the case, *don't stop!* Keep doing your journal. You never go beyond being in relationship to your body. You need to keep paying attention to your eating. If your food starts getting sloppy, if your energy changes, if you start getting restless, if you slip into la-la land, if you start to double-book your appointments or forget things and become short-tempered, your journal will be there to help you. Your faithful friend will remind you about your special biochemistry. When you look in your journal, you may find that your food is stable and other factors in your life are affecting how you feel. The journal will allow you to either pinpoint biochemical factors or exclude them. Either way, you remain a step ahead of the game.

HOLDING IT

Let's review the key points you want to remember.

Continue Your Food Journal No Matter What

Your journal is the cornerstone of your recovery. Doing the journal keeps you *in relationship* to your body. It reminds you of the connection between what you eat and how you feel. The journal keeps you honest and rigorous about what you want. The journal reinforces living consciously. The journal, as you may have guessed by now, is about far more than your food.

Maintain Your Blood Sugar Level

Stay steady and clear. Always have breakfast. Eat three meals a day at regular intervals. Eat from the right side of the carbohydrate continuum. Stay in good company by eating brown things and green things. Choose foods with the lowest impact value— the least sugar and the most fiber.

Enhance Your Serotonin Level

Eat protein at each meal. Make sure that enough tryptophan is swimming around in your blood. Have your potato (without any protein) three hours after your protein meal to boost little tryptophan into your brain. Don't be tricked into thinking that this is too simple to work. Pay attention to the effects and you will remain a believer.

Enhance Your Beta-endorphin Level

Reduce or eliminate sugars and white things to minimize the beta-endorphin priming that comes with a "hit" of sugar. Make life changes to increase the behaviors and activities (listed below) that evoke or support the production of your own beta-endorphin in a steady and consistent way.

Remember that your body was designed for the release of beta-endorphin to support "the good life." Let's list the things besides alcohol, drugs, and sugars that evoke beta-endorphin.

- Meditation
- Yoga
- Exercise
- Prayer
- Music
- Eating food that tastes good
- Orgasm
- Cooking
- Dancing
- Working in the garden
- Listening to inspirational talks
- Being with the people, puppies, or kitties that you love

Most of the things on this list have been talked about in the scientific literature. There are actually scientific articles about the beta-endorphin effect of exercise, meditation, music, yoga, prayer, inspirational talks, sex, and palatable food. And no, "food that tastes good" does not just mean sugar or fat. It just means food that tastes good in the mouth.

While the beta-endorphin response to these behaviors is documented in scientific journals, I imagine that your own experience can easily confirm their findings. I added dancing and being with puppies and kitties because the response sure feels like beta-endorphin. It does seem interesting that the things that are associated with being "high on life" are the beta-endorphin things. It may well be that we were given beta-endorphin to push us to do the things associated with wholeness and happiness.

You may wonder if doing these things will raise your beta-endorphin, create downregulation, and then leave you stranded if you can't keep it up. I don't think it works that way. Supporting your body's own production of beta-endorphin with things like meditation, prayer, and exercise enhances the production in a slow, steady rate over time. It does not create those dreaded spikes. I call these "soft BE." Your neurotransmitters and neuro-receptors stay balanced the way they are designed to. People who achieve an integrated and focused life, a life with balanced and integrated biochemistry, feel good.

You are learning that the beta-endorphin story is bigger than food.

Enhance Your Dopamine Level

"Your *what* level?" you are probably asking. Dopamine is a brain chemical like serotonin and beta-endorphin. I didn't include it in our earlier discussion of brain chemicals, because in your early recovery, I want to keep things as simple as possible. We are just learning about dopamine. Bart Hoebel, the scientist I referred to earlier, is doing some very intriguing work on the connection between sugar and dopamine. I am quite sure this will be a topic for my next book. When dopamine is present at an optimal level, you feel motivated, creative, joyful about life, and sexually alive. Many sugar-sensitive people have discovered that things like diet pills, caffeine, diet soda, speed, cocaine, and danger can create these feelings by waking up dopamine. Learning to raise dopamine without falling into an addictive "going for the rush" trap requires skill and maturity in recovery. I see dopamine as the brain chemical for Step 7 work.

But you can get the benefits long before you have all the science of dopamine. Enhancing your dopamine level in a healthy way comes with exercise and meditation. These activities quiet the addictive spiking that you have used in the past to feel uplifted. You want life without the spike. Moving and being still is the antidote. All sugar-sensitive people need to move. Even if you start with just a five-minute walk, you will want to include this in your program. If you are at the other end of the scale, doing four hours of exercise a day, you will want to find ways to be fit without the potential for addiction brought on by overstimulating your beta-endorphin and dopamine.

Besides needing to move, you need to be quiet. Meditation will quiet you. The meditation you do does not need to be formal or complicated. It does not need to be the kind of practice you may associate with Buddhism or the Far East or the New Age. The type of meditation I am suggesting is different from prayer or listening to a relaxation tape. This is about being still. Just sit quietly without distraction. If the dog whines, put the dog in the crate and close the door. Put the cat in the other room. Ask your husband or partner to be with the kids. Turn off the phone if there's one in the room. You need alone time and quiet time.

The best times for meditation are early morning and at 8:00 p.m. Early morning will create the most focus because your natural beta-endorphin level is the highest, and higher beta-endorphin will create soft dopamine. Remember that all the brain chemicals are connected. Enhancing one can help the others. At 8:00 p.m.

your natural beta-endorphin level is the lowest, so you will get the biggest effect—the stilling and quieting of a jumping brain.

DISCERNING FOOD ISSUES FROM LIFE ISSUES

After you have followed this program for a while, you will begin to know clearly and quickly which physical symptoms are connected to your food. Certainly not all of them will be. But the joy for you will be to know how to differentiate. If you are feeling out of sorts you will learn to recognize when your feelings can be traced to a withdrawal from the crazy dessert you had yesterday. The disturbing feelings that are simply part of withdrawal will pass and life will return to normal.

As you have longer periods of time in which your food is stable, you'll also be able to distinguish real-life situations you need to deal with. Your marriage may be falling apart but you never looked at the reality because you were always medicated with sugar or alcohol. Or your life may not be what you want it to be and you never saw it before because of too many hot fudge sundaes. Or your depression may be creeping back. But you will know so much more about the biochemistry of what is happening, you will be ready with the options for responding to these issues.

Issues like these are life questions we all must face. There are answers. There are people who can share the journey with you. Discovering these questions will enrich your life and deepen who you are.

THERE'S NO SUCH THING AS PERFECTION

"Progress not perfection" is a core Twelve-Step slogan and one that is particularly useful for doing food recovery. You cannot ever have a perfect journey with food. Life is too complex and textured for perfection. The real perfection you will attain is the joy and confidence you will feel about mastering your "crazy" body chemistry. When I talk about radiance, I am talking about a way of being in the world that reflects your core self. Radiance moves you to humor, tenderness, enjoyment, and delight. Radiance urges you to meditate, laugh, dance, pray, sing, paint, read, run, seek good food, intimacy, and good company, and connect to meaning. As you step into your new way of being in the world, you will no longer settle for mere relief from pain or problems. You will want more than that.

You will find that all the work you have done with that funny little food journal has prepared you for taking these next steps, for achieving radiance. The art of paying attention, having a plan, and doing one step at a time is an invaluable ally for your future. What you have been practicing these past months is about far more than food. This journey is much bigger than just changing what you are eating. As you heal your food, you are healing the deepest part of who you are. Changing your relationship to food means changing your relationship to yourself, to your ways of nourishment, and your connection to your birthright. You are a bright, creative, sensitive, and awesome person. These too are inherited benefits of sugar sensitivity.

We've talked a lot about the downside of sugar sensitivity, but the other side of sugar sensitivity is a special kind of awareness, intuition, and compassion that comes with the very same biochemistry. Being born with lower beta-endorphin means you are less insulated. You do feel pain more intensely, but you also feel joy more deeply. You know in every part of who you are that something creative, awesome, and magical is waiting for you. The same molecules that once sang for sugar will now sing for radiance.

As you come into balance, you can shape your own direction rather than being driven by biochemical circumstances. You feel empowered to make changes in your life and to control what is happening to you. What seemed like a story about food is really a story about possibility. Fear of being a bag lady or a wino on the street has given way to confidence and opportunity. And it all started with eating breakfast.

APPENDIX

DETOXIFICATION FROM ALCOHOL

Be tender with yourself as you look at your relationship to alcohol. If you have a problem with alcohol, you probably have had all sorts of people who have been far from tender with you. No doubt you have been criticized, shamed, fought with, talked to, cajoled, bargained with, or argued with. In fact, if someone around you criticizes your drinking, it is one of the most reliable indicators that you have a problem with alcohol. People who do not have a problem with alcohol do not evoke pain, frustration, or concern about drinking in the people around them.

Take a quiet look at your alcohol use. You don't have to admit you have a problem, you don't have to surrender anything. Your own commitment and experience will guide you in this process. Honesty about your relationship to alcohol is hard because the very nature of the disease of alcoholism is denial. Do this review in the privacy of your own home or office and give yourself absolute discretion over whether you share your findings with anyone at this time. If privacy supports your honesty, embrace it. If sharing serves you better, find a trusted friend to help you ask these questions. The very best alternative is a friend in recovery.

What is very surprising is that people who do not have a problem with drinking don't feel bad about it. They don't feel guilty. We talk a lot about the denial of alcoholism. I believe denial is the response that emerges when people are made to feel defensive about their behaviors. When there is no reason to be defensive, people are remarkably on target about what is going on with them. Take away the shame or the judgment and they can assess their problems pretty clearly.

"Oh, come on," you say. "Everyone does that!" Everyone doesn't do this. People who don't have a problem with alcohol are not inclined to want more when they feel bad. Having a problem with alcohol or alcoholism is defined as "continued use of alcohol despite adverse consequences." When a non–problem drinker has an adverse consequence from drinking, she stops. She will make the connection between feeling bad and alcohol. A problem drinker doesn't see this connection.

Not making the connection is not about being stubborn or stupid or even about willful denial. Not making the connection between drinking and feeling bad is about chemical changes in the brain that alter the parts of the brain that form judgment by making a connection between cause and effect. The parts of the brain that are responsible for saying, "Hey, this made me feel bad. I don't think I want more," don't work properly.

Not making the connection creates a vicious cycle. In the problem drinker's mind, the alcohol actually makes her feel better, so she drinks more. Her opinion is confirmed when the alcohol triggers a beta-endorphin release of euphoric feelings. This reaction is why everyone drinks—the effect is nice. The sugar-sensitive person feels especially good because alcohol causes an even greater beta-endorphin response in her brain. She feels far better than other people do when they drink.

But the next morning she is hung over, a feeling that comes from withdrawal. All the beta-endorphin receptors that were stimulated, or primed, by yesterday's alcohol use are screaming for more. That morning-after feeling of wanting to do *anything* to feel better is so easily taken care of by having a drink. So she does. Relief comes. Blessed, sweet relief. And with her "adverse consequences" switch turned off, the problem drinker's natural response is to feel that having a quick one is a reasonable and logical way to take care of bad feelings. She doesn't know that difficulty with alcohol is creeping up on her.

You may have this same blind spot. How can you know if you have a problem? Let's go back to the questions on pages 183–84 Taken together, these questions form the CAGE, which stands for:

C—CRITICIZED
A—ANNOYED
G—GUILTY
E—EYE-OPENER

Now, let's look at each question individually.

- **Have you ever felt you should cut down on your drinking?** Not a hard one. People usually know the answer to this right away. Yes or no. No cheating or fudging. If cutting down is even a passing thought, answer this one yes.
- **Have people ever Annoyed you by criticizing your drinking?** Okay, be honest now. Ever? Think about those times when you held your tongue or wanted to smack someone for making a comment about your drinking. Think of the fights you've had with your spouse about it. Answer honestly.
- **Have you ever felt bad or Guilty about your drinking?** This question is pretty straightforward.
- **Have you ever had a drink first thing in the morning (an Eye-opener) to steady your nerves or to get rid of a hangover?**

A score of even one is a warning sign about a problem.

Remember the meaning of CAGE. Let yourself think about this for a while. One of two things will happen. You might begin working very hard to say, "Naw, I don't really feel guilty about my drinking." This is an example of denial creeping in and wrapping its deadly little body around your neck. Just pay attention. Consider whether you are getting further away from your relationship to your body and your own inner wisdom.

The other thing that might happen is you may be jostled into realizing that you have a problem with alcohol. If you decide that you would like to stop drinking, there are a number of factors to take into consideration before you do. First, you'll need to estimate how severe a withdrawal you will have based on the frequency and volume of your drinking. You'll need to honestly and accurately figure out how much alcohol you consume in a week. You can do this by recording your alcohol consumption right in your food journal. Do this for a week and then take an honest look at the frequency and amount of your drinking. Calculate the number of drinks you have in a day or a week. A drink is 4 ounces of wine, one beer, or 1 ounce of hard liquor. So if you have three 6-ounce glasses of wine (18 ounces), this would be the equivalent of 4.5 drinks.

After you know where you now stand, you can start to plan your detox process. Just as in your detox from sugars, you will want to determine your style for making change. You can either taper down and then stop or you can stop all at once. Most people find it much easier to go for sobriety all at once. You don't have to be making decisions about how much, when, where, with whom all of the time. You can focus on one decision only—the decision not to drink.

It will be important for you to have some sort of support as you make the change. Do not stop drinking without telling anyone what you are doing. Find someone who has been through alcohol detox. Talk to that person. Alcoholics Anonymous (AA) can be a wonderful support because everyone there has been through this process. The only requirement for going to AA is a desire to stop drinking. You don't have to be an alcoholic. You don't have to sign up, you don't have to agree with the program, you don't have to do it any particular way. You don't even have to talk at the meeting. You can sit quietly in the back and slip out quickly anytime you want.

AA can give you a lifeline to others who know about recovery. They can provide you with a road map and concrete suggestions about how to handle what you are feeling. If you go to a meeting and don't like it, don't assume that you won't like a different meeting. Some meetings are boring, some are abusive, and most are profoundly supportive and life-giving.

If you are not comfortable at meetings, find at least one person to support you in your alcohol detox. Do not expect your spouse, partner, daughter, or son to be your primary support. They are too closely involved. Find at least one person who has been there. Talk about what you are doing. Tell your story. Get books about recovery. Go to a treatment professional.

If you plan to stop drinking all at once, you must have medical supervision for your detox if any of the following are true for you:

1. If you have a history of blood pressure that is higher than 140/90.
2. If you have drunk more than a six-pack of beer, more than six 4-ounce glasses of wine or more than 8 ounces (half a pint) of liquor daily for over a year.
3. If you have had prior withdrawal symptoms, such as depression or agitation.
4. If you have ever had seizures for any reason, and in particular if you have had alcohol DTs.
5. If you are using any other (either illegal or prescription) drugs in combination with the alcohol. This particularly includes benzodiazepines such as Valium, Librium, or Xanax.

Withdrawal from significant or long-standing alcohol use can be a serious process. Keep yourself safe as you make this change. You are taking a very important and brave step. Withdrawal symptoms can include depression, insomnia, sweating, tremulousness, agitation, irritability, and brain fog. Withdrawal usually starts four to six hours after you usually have your alcohol. If you drink every day at 6 p.m., you will begin to experience discomfort that evening. If you have been a heavy drinker, your doctor may prescribe short-term medication which will minimize the possibility of having seizures during detox.

Making the food changes in preparation for going off alcohol will greatly enhance the likelihood that you can achieve and maintain long-term sobriety. The first week you stop drinking, increase your vitamin and fruit intake. If you feel edgy during the day, have an additional ½ teaspoon of the B-complex liquid. (Don't have it in the evening, though; it will keep you up.) We encourage our clients to have two or three bananas a day for that first week. You can add one to your power shake and then use them as a snack later in the day. Make sure you have a baked potato before you go to bed. It will help your serotonin function and will support the normalization of your sleep patterns.

The clients in my clinic cannot believe what a difference it makes to have done the food plan first. They have fewer withdrawal symptoms, very little craving, and feel better than they have in years. This food plan can support the power of your commitment.

GLOSSARY

Abundance model
An approach to healing based on "adding" rather than "taking away." This method helps the individual have a greater sense of possibility, more confidence about options, and a sense of hope. The abundance model reinforces the belief that each person knows how to find healing and only needs the appropriate tools to find a healing path.

Addiction
Compulsive use of a substance or behavior characterized by an increasing tolerance for that substance or behavior and the symptoms of physiological withdrawal when the substance or behavior is stopped.

Adrenal fatigue
A progressive physical response by the adrenal glands to long-term stress resulting from difficult situations, the use of alcohol or drugs, or certain dietary patterns, especially the frequent use of sugar. Negatively affects the rapidity and effectiveness of the

body's normal ability to regulate blood sugar levels. Adrenal fatigue exacerbates addiction.

Antidepressant medications
Psychotherapeutic drugs designed to minimize depression by increasing the availability of serotonin or other neurotransmitters implicated in the physiology of depression.

Beta-endorphin
A brain chemical (specifically, a neurotransmitter) responsible for modulating emotional and physical pain. Contributes to feelings of self-esteem, euphoria, and emotional confidence.

Brown things
Whole-grain complex carbohydrates retaining high levels of fiber. They include such things as whole grains, and breads and cereals made with whole grains, brown rice, potatoes, lentils, nuts, and beans. See page 165 for a list of brown things.

Carbohydrate continuum
A chart showing the relative complexity of different carbohydrates ranging from simple sugars to wood. See page 151.

Complex carbohydrates
Carbohydrates having more than three simple sugars strung together. They include starches, brown things, and green things.

Covert sugars
Sugars that are "hidden" in processed foods. They include such things as high-fructose corn syrup, maltodextrin, raisin paste, etc.

Deprivation model
An approach to healing that requires the individual to give up things. Assumes that the person is unable to make change without rules and restrictions.

Downregulation
A process in the brain by which the number of neuroreceptors for a certain brain chemical decreases to compensate for an increase in the number of neurotransmitters carrying that chemical.

Dr. Jekyll/Mr. Hyde syndrome
The emotional and physical Ping-Pong arising from untreated sugar sensitivity. Feelings and behaviors are erratic and unpredictable and contribute to greatly decreased effectiveness in dealing with the world.

Endogenous opioids
Neurotransmitters produced within the brain that act as natural painkillers for both physical and emotional pain. Beta-endorphin is a key endogenous opioid.

Food journal
A written log that records the amount and type of food eaten, the date and time, and the physical and emotional feelings.

Green things
Complex carbohydrates, including green, yellow, white, purple, and red vegetables.

Hypoglycemia
Low blood sugar resulting from a number of causes, such as not eating regularly or eating foods high in sugars. Sugar-sensitive people are more vulnerable to hypoglycemia because they are thought to have an exaggerated insulin response to sweet foods. (See *Low blood sugar*.)

Impulse control
The ability to "just say no." The gap between your intention and your actually doing something. Mediated by the level of serotonin in your brain. Low serotonin results in low impulse control and vice versa.

Isolation distress
Emotional pain induced from being separated from a loving and supportive environment. Feelings of isolation distress increase as a person's level of beta-endorphin drops and decrease as beta-endorphin rises.

Low blood sugar
A physical state in which the amount of glucose in the blood drops and creates such symptoms as fatigue, irritability, loss of concentration, and emotional vulnerability.

Naltrexone
A drug that blocks the painkilling effect of opioid drugs such as heroin.

Neuroreceptors
Specialized receiving centers on the cell that are coded to accept their matched neurotransmitters and send the appropriate message through the cell.

Neurotransmitters
Brain chemicals responsible for sending specialized messages from one brain cell to another. This book talks about the neurotransmitters serotonin, beta-endorphin, and dopamine.

Overt sugars
Sugars that are clearly associated with being sweet, such as table sugar, honey, syrup, and the sugars found in ice cream, cookies, cake, or soda pop.

Priming
The biochemical activation of the beta-endorphin system by one drug, which initiates craving for more of the same or for a drug with a similar effect. For example, eating sugar makes you want more sugar. Eating sugar can also make you want alcohol.

PMS (Premenstrual Syndrome)
In the period prior to menstruation, beta-endorphin levels plummet, cravings for sweets increase, and difficult physical and emotional symptoms are made worse.

Power bar
A nutritional food designed to provide quick energy. Generally billed as "low-fat," power bars are often high in multiple sugars.

Relapse
A return to compulsive or addictive behavior. See also *Slip*.

Reuptake pump
A mechanism that acts like a vacuum cleaner to recycle used neurotransmitters.

Serotonin
A neurotransmitter responsible for mood and for impulsive and compulsive behavior.

Simple carbohydrates
Sugars such as the monosaccharides: glucose, fructose, galactose, and the disaccharides: maltose, sucrose, lactose.

Slip
Short-term flirting with compulsive or addictive behavior. If a "slip" continues for more than a few days, it progresses into "relapse."

Starches
A long chain of hundreds of glucose molecules linked together. Starches are found in grains, beans, and vegetables.

Sugar sensitivity
A biochemical condition creating puzzling physical and emotional ups and downs. Sugar sensitivity is characterized by volatile

blood sugar responses, a low level of serotonin, a low level of beta-endorphin, and a heightened response to the pain-numbing effects of sugars.

Upregulation
A process in the brain by which the number of neuroreceptors for a certain brain chemical increase to compensate for a reduction in the number of neurotransmitters carrying that chemical.

White things
Foods made from refined grains and simple starches without fiber. Includes such things as white breads, pasta, white rice, and potatoes without the skin.

Withdrawal
A physiological response within the brain when receptor sites have become adapted to a certain level of neurotransmitters and "complain" when that level is reduced. Withdrawal symptoms can include fatigue, irritability, nausea, sleeplessness, headaches, constipation, and diarrhea.

BIBLIOGRAPHY

Akkok, F., et al. Naloxone persistently modifies water-intake. *Pharmacol Biochem Behav*, 1988. 29(2): 331–34.

Anderson, I. M., et al. Dieting reduces plasma tryptophan and alters brain 5-HT function in women. *Psychol Med*, 1990. 20(4): 785–91.

Angelogianni, P., and C. Gianoulakis. Ontogeny of the beta-endorphin response to stress in the rat: role of the pituitary and the hypothalamus. *Neuroendocrinology*, 1989. 50(4): 372–81.

———. Prenatal exposure to ethanol alters the ontogeny of the beta-endorphin response to stress. *Alcohol Clin Exp Res*, 1989. 13(4): 564–71.

Avena, N. M., and B. G. Hoebel. A diet promoting sugar dependency causes behavioral cross-sensitization to a low dose of amphetamine. *Neuroscience*, 2003. 122(1): 17–20.

———. Amphetamine-sensitized rats show sugar-induced hyperactivity (cross-sensitization) and sugar hyperphagia. *Pharmacol Biochem Behav*, 2003. 74(3): 635–39.

Avena, N. M., K. A. Long, and B. G. Hoebel. Sugar-dependent rats show enhanced responding for sugar after abstinence: evidence of a sugar deprivation effect. *Physiol Behav*, 2005. 84(3): 359–62.

Avena, N. M., et al. Sugar-dependent rats show enhanced intake of unsweetened ethanol. *Alcohol*, 2004. 34(2–3): 203–9.

Avena, N. M., et al. Sucrose sham feeding on a binge schedule releases accumbens dopamine repeatedly and eliminates the acetylcholine satiety response. *Neuroscience*, 2006. 139(3): 813–20.

Beczkowska, I. W., W. D. Bowen, and R. J. Bodnar. Central opioid receptor subtype antagonists differentially alter sucrose and deprivation-induced water intake in rats. *Brain Res*, 1992. 589(2): 291–301.

Bencherif, B., et al. Regional mu-opioid receptor binding in insular cortex is decreased in bulimia nervosa and correlates inversely with fasting behavior. *J Nucl Med*, 2005. 46(8): 1349–51.

Blass, E. M., and A. Shah. Pain-reducing properties of sucrose in human newborns. *Chem Senses*, 1995. 20(1): 29–35.

Blass, E. M., and L. B. Watt. Suckling- and sucrose-induced analgesia in human newborns. *Pain*, 1999. 83(3): 611–23.

Blass, E., E. Fitzgerald, and P. Kehoe. Interactions between sucrose, pain and isolation distress. *Pharmacol Biochem Behav*, 1987. 26(3): 483–89.

Blass, E. M., et al. Separation of opioid from nonopioid mediation of affect in neonatal rats: nonopioid mechanisms mediate maternal contact influences. *Behav Neurosci*, 1990. 104(4): 625–36.

Brunani, A., et al. Influence of insulin on beta-endorphin plasma levels in obese and normal weight subjects. *Int J Obes Relat Metab Disord*, 1996. 20(8): 710–14.

Bujatti, M., and P. Riederer. Serotonin, noradrenaline, dopamine metabolites in transcendental meditation-technique. *J Neural Transm*, 1976. 39(3): 257–67.

Carrillo, C. A., et al. A high-fat meal or injection of lipids stimulates ethanol intake. *Alcohol*, 2004. 34(2–3): 197–202.

Chang, G. Q., et al. Effect of ethanol on hypothalamic opioid peptides, enkephalin, and dynorphin: relationship with circulating triglycerides. *Alcohol Clin Exp Res*, 2007. 31(2): 249–59.

Christie, M. J., and G. B. Chesher. Physical dependence on physiologically released endogenous opiates. *Life Sci*, 1982. 30(14): 1173–77.

Cleary, J., et al. Naloxone effects on sucrose-motivated behavior. *Psychopharmacology* (Berl), 1996. 126(2): 110–14.

Colantuoni, C., et al. Evidence that intermittent, excessive sugar intake causes endogenous opioid dependence. *Obes Res*, 2002. 10(6): 478–88.

Colantuoni, C., et al. Excessive sugar intake alters binding to dopamine and mu-opioid receptors in the brain. *Neuroreport*, 2001. 12(16): 3549–52.

Cronin, A., et al. Opioid inhibition of rapid eye movement sleep by a specific mu receptor agonist. Br J Anaesth, 1995. 74(2): 188–92.

Czirr, S. A., et al. Selected opioids modify intake of sweetened ethanol solution among female rats. Alcohol, 1987. 4(3): 157–60.

Czirr, S. A., and L. D. Reid. Demonstrating morphine's potentiating effects on sucrose-intake. Brain Res Bull, 1986. 17(5): 639–42.

Dai, X., J. Thavundayil, and C. Gianoulakis. Differences in the peripheral levels of beta-endorphin in response to alcohol and stress as a function of alcohol dependence and family history of alcoholism. Alcohol Clin Exp Res, 2005. 29(11): 1965–75.

d'Anci, K. E., and R. B. Kanarek. Naltrexone antagonism of morphine antinociception in sucrose- and chow-fed rats. Nutr Neurosci, 2004. 7(1): 57–61.

d'Anci, K. E., A. V. Gerstein, and R. B. Kanarek. Long-term voluntary access to running wheels decreases kappa-opioid antinociception. Pharmacol Biochem Behav, 2000. 66(2): 343–46.

d'Anci, K. E., R. B. Kanarek, and R. Marks-Kaufman. Duration of sucrose availability differentially alters morphine-induced analgesia in rats. Pharmacol Biochem Behav, 1996. 54(4): 693–97.

Davidson, R. Meditation and neuroplasticity: training your brain. Interview by Bonnie J. Horrigan. Explore (NY), 2005. 1(5): 380–88.

Davidson, R. J., et al. Alterations in brain and immune function produced by mindfulness meditation. Psychosom Med, 2003. 65(4): 564–70.

de Waele, J. P., and C. Gianoulakis. Effects of ethanol on the brain beta-endorphin system in inbred strains of mice with variable preference for ethanol solutions: in vitro study. Prog Clin Biol Res, 1990. 328: 315–18.

———. Characterization of the mu and delta opioid receptors in the brain of the C57BL/6 and DBA/2 mice, selected for their differences in voluntary ethanol consumption. Alcohol Clin Exp Res, 1997. 21(4): 754–62.

de Waele, J. P., K. Kiianmaa, and C. Gianoulakis. Distribution of the mu and delta opioid binding sites in the brain of the alcohol-preferring AA and alcohol-avoiding ANA lines of rats. J Pharmacol Exp Ther, 1995. 275(1): 518–27.

de Waele, J. P., D. N. Papachristou, and C. Gianoulakis. The alcohol-preferring C57BL/6 mice present an enhanced sensitivity of the hypothalamic beta-endorphin system to ethanol than the alcohol-avoiding DBA/2 mice. J Pharmacol Exp Ther, 1992. 261(2): 788–94.

Drewnowski, A. Metabolic determinants of binge eating. *Addict Behav*, 1995. 20(6): 733–45.

Drewnowski, A., and M. R. Greenwood. Cream and sugar: human preferences for high-fat foods. *Physiol Behav*, 1983. 30(4): 629–33.

Drewnowski, A., et al. Taste responses and preferences for sweet high-fat foods: evidence for opioid involvement. *Physiol Behav*, 1992. 51(2): 371–79.

Drewnowski, A., et al. Naloxone, an opiate blocker, reduces the consumption of sweet high-fat foods in obese and lean female binge eaters. *Am J Clin Nutr*, 1995. 61(6): 1206–12.

Drewnowski, A., et al. Food preferences in human obesity: carbohydrates versus fats. *Appetite*, 1992. 18(3): 207–21.

Elfhag, K., and C. Erlanson-Albertsson. Sweet and fat taste preference in obesity have different associations with personality and eating behavior. *Physiol Behav*, 2006. 88(1–2): 61–66.

Erlanson-Albertsson, C. [Sugar triggers our reward-system. Sweets release opiates which stimulate the appetite for sucrose—insulin can depress it]. *Lakartidningen*, 2005. 102(21): 1620–22, 1625, 1627.

Erlanson-Albertsson, C., and J. Mei. The effect of low carbohydrate on energy metabolism. *Int J Obes* (Lond), 2005. 29 Suppl 2: S26–30.

Fantino, M., J. Hosotte, and M. Apfelbaum. An opioid antagonist, naltrexone, reduces preference for sucrose in humans. *Am J Physiol*, 1986. 251(1 Pt 2): R91–96.

Fernstrom, J. D. Effects on the diet on brain neurotransmitters. *Metabolism*, 1977. 26(2): 207–23.

———. Tryptophan, serotonin and carbohydrate appetite: will the real carbohydrate craver please stand up! *J Nutr*, 1988. 118(11): 1417–19.

Fernstrom, J. D., and D. V. Faller. Neutral amino acids in the brain: changes in response to food ingestion. *J Neurochem*, 1978. 30(6): 1531–38.

Fernstrom, J. D., and R. J. Wurtman. Control of brain serotonin levels by the diet. *Adv Biochem Psychopharmacol*, 1974. 11(0): 133–42.

Fernstrom, M. H., and J. D. Fernstrom. Brain tryptophan concentrations and serotonin synthesis remain responsive to food consumption after the ingestion of sequential meals. *Am J Clin Nutr*, 1995. 61(2): 312–19.

Fullerton, D. T., et al. Sugar, opioids and binge eating. *Brain Res Bull*, 1985. 14(6): 673–80.

Genazzani, A. R., et al. Central deficiency of beta-endorphin in alcohol addicts. *J Clin Endocrinol Metab*, 1982. 55(3): 583–86.

Gentry, R. T., and V. P. Dole. Why does a sucrose choice reduce the consumption of alcohol in C57BL/6J mice? *Life Sci*, 1987. 40(22): 2191–94.

Giannini, A. J., et al. Symptoms of premenstrual syndrome as a function of beta-endorphin: two subtypes. *Prog Neuropsychopharmacol Biol Psychiatry*, 1994. 18(2): 321–27.

Gianoulakis, C. Long-term ethanol alters the binding of 3H-opiates to brain membranes. *Life Sci*, 1983. 33(8): 725–33.

———. The effect of ethanol on the biosynthesis and regulation of opioid peptides. *Experientia*, 1989. 45(5): 428–35.

———. Characterization of the effects of acute ethanol administration on the release of beta-endorphin peptides by the rat hypothalamus. *Eur J Pharmacol*, 1990. 180(1): 21–29.

———. Endogenous opioids and excessive alcohol consumption. *J Psychiatry Neurosci*, 1993. 18(4): 148–56.

———. Implications of endogenous opioids and dopamine in alcoholism: human and basic science studies. *Alcohol Alcohol Suppl*, 1996. 1: 33–42.

———. Influence of the endogenous opioid system on high alcohol consumption and genetic predisposition to alcoholism. *J Psychiatry Neurosci*, 2001. 26(4): 304–18.

———. Endogenous opioids and addiction to alcohol and other drugs of abuse. *Curr Top Med Chem*, 2004. 4(1): 39–50.

Gianoulakis, C., and J. P. de Waele. Genetics of alcoholism: role of the endogenous opioid system. *Metab Brain Dis*, 1994. 9(2): 105–31.

Gianoulakis, C., J. P. de Waele, and K. Kiianmaa. Differences in the brain and pituitary beta-endorphin system between the alcohol-preferring AA and alcohol-avoiding ANA rats. *Alcohol Clin Exp Res*, 1992. 16(3): 453–59.

Gianoulakis, C., J. P. de Waele, and J. Thavundayil. Implication of the endogenous opioid system in excessive ethanol consumption. *Alcohol*, 1996. 13(1): 19–23.

Goldman, J. A., et al. Behavioral effects of sucrose on preschool children. *J Abnorm Child Psychol*, 1986. 14(4): 565–77.

Gosnell, B. A. Central structures involved in opioid-induced feeding. *Fed Proc*, 1987. 46(1): 163–67.

Gosnell, B. A. Involvement of mu opioid receptors in the amygdala in the control of feeding. *Neuropharmacology*, 1988. 27(3): 319–26.

———. Sucrose intake predicts rate of acquisition of cocaine self-administration. *Psychopharmacology* (Berl), 2000. 149(3): 286–92.

———. Sucrose intake enhances behavioral sensitization produced by cocaine. *Brain Res*, 2005. 1031(2): 194–201.

Gosnell, B. A., and D. D. Krahn. The effects of continuous morphine infusion on diet selection and body weight. *Physiol Behav*, 1993. 54(5): 853–59.

———. Taste and diet preferences as predictors of drug self-administration. *NIDA Res Monogr*, 1998. 169: 154–75.

Gosnell, B. A., and M. J. Majchrzak. Effects of a selective mu opioid receptor agonist and naloxone on the intake of sodium chloride solutions. *Psychopharmacology* (Berl), 1990. 100(1): 66–71.

Gosnell, B. A., D. D. Krahn, and M.J. Majchrzak. The effects of morphine on diet selection are dependent upon baseline diet preferences. *Pharmacol Biochem Behav*, 1990. 37(2): 207–12.

Gosnell, B. A., A. S. Levine, and J. E. Morley. The effects of aging on opioid modulation of feeding in rats. *Life Sci*, 1983. 32(24): 2793–99.

Gosnell, B. A., M. J. Majchrzak, and D. D. Krahn. Effects of preferential delta and kappa opioid receptor agonists on the intake of hypotonic saline. *Physiol Behav*, 1990. 47(3): 601–3.

Gosnell, B. A., J. E. Morley, and A. S. Levine. Opioid-induced feeding: localization of sensitive brain sites. *Brain Res*, 1986. 369(1–2): 177–84.

Grau, J. W., et al. Long-term stress-induced analgesia and activation of the opiate system. *Science*, 1981. 213(4514): 1409–11.

Holt, S. H., et al. A satiety index of common foods. *Eur J Clin Nutr*, 1995. 49(9): 675–90.

Holter, S. M., et al. Kappa-opioid receptors and relapse-like drinking in long-term ethanol-experienced rats. *Psychopharmacology* (Berl), 2000. 153(1): 93–102.

Hutchison, W. D., C. Gianoulakis, and H. Kalant. Effects of ethanol withdrawal on beta-endorphin levels in rat brain and pituitary. *Pharmacol Biochem Behav*, 1988. 30(4): 933–39.

Israel, K. D., et al. Serum uric acid, inorganic phosphorus, and glutamic-oxalacetic transaminase and blood pressure in carbohydrate-sensitive adults consuming three different levels of sucrose. *Ann Nutr Metab*, 1983. 27(5): 425–35.

Jenkins, D. J., et al. Slowly digested carbohydrate food improves impaired carbohydrate tolerance in patients with cirrhosis. *Clin Sci* (Lond), 1984. 66(6): 649–57.

Jewett, D. C., M. K. Grace, and A. S. Levine. Chronic sucrose ingestion enhances mu-opioid discriminative stimulus effects. *Brain Res*, 2005. 1050(1–2): 48–52.

Kampov-Polevoy, A. B., J. C. Garbutt, and D. Janowsky. Evidence of preference for a high-concentration sucrose solution in alcoholic men. *Am J Psychiatry*, 1997. 154(2): 269–70.

———. Association between preference for sweets and excessive alcohol intake: a review of animal and human studies. *Alcohol Alcohol*, 1999. 34(3): 386–95.

Kampov-Polevoy, A. B., J. C. Garbutt, and E. Khalitov. Family history of alcoholism and response to sweets. *Alcohol Clin Exp Res*, 2003. 27(11): 1743–49.

Kampov-Polevoy, A. B., et al. Sweet liking and family history of alcoholism in hospitalized alcoholic and non-alcoholic patients. *Alcohol Alcohol*, 2001. 36(2): 165–70.

Kampov-Polevoy, A. B., et al. Sweet liking, novelty seeking, and gender predict alcoholic status. *Alcohol Clin Exp Res*, 2004. 28(9): 1291–98.

Kampov-Polevoy, A. B., et al. Sweet preference predicts mood altering effect of and impaired control over eating sweet foods. *Eat Behav*, 2006. 7(3): 181–87.

Kanarek, R. B., B. A. Homoleski, and C. Wiatr. Intake of a palatable sucrose solution modifies the actions of spiradoline, a kappa opioid receptor agonist, on analgesia and feeding behavior in male and female rats. *Pharmacol Biochem Behav*, 2000. 65(1): 97–104.

Kanarek, R. B., S. Mandillo, and C. Wiatr. Chronic sucrose intake augments antinociception induced by injections of mu but not kappa opioid receptor agonists into the periaqueductal gray matter in male and female rats. *Brain Res*, 2001. 920(1–2): 97–105.

Kanarek, R. B., et al. Dietary modulation of mu and kappa opioid receptor-mediated analgesia. *Pharmacol Biochem Behav*, 1997. 58(1): 43–49.

Kanarek, R. B., et al. Dietary influences on morphine-induced analgesia in rats. *Pharmacol Biochem Behav*, 1991. 38(3): 681–84.

Kehoe, P., and E. M. Blass. Opioid-mediation of separation distress in 10-day-old rats: reversal of stress with maternal stimuli. *Dev Psychobiol*, 1986. 19(4): 385–98.

Knapp, D. J., et al. Ultrasonic vocalization behavior differs between lines of ethanol-preferring and nonpreferring rats. *Alcohol Clin Exp Res,* 1997. 21(7): 1232–40.

Koob, G. F. Neurobiology of addiction. Toward the development of new therapies. *Ann N Y Acad Sci,* 2000. 909: 170–85.

Krahn, D. D., et al. Caffeine consumption in patients with eating disorders. *Hosp Community Psychiatry,* 1991. 42(3): 313–15.

Kunz, J., Ice cream preference: gender differences in taste and quality. *Percept Mot Skills,* 1993. 77(3 Pt 2): 1097–98.

Kuzmin, A., et al. Enhancement of morphine self-administration in drug naive, inbred strains of mice by acute emotional stress. *Eur Neuropsychopharmacol,* 1996. 6(1): 63–68.

Laeng, B., K. C. Berridge, and C. M. Butter. Pleasantness of a sweet taste during hunger and satiety: effects of gender and "sweet tooth." *Appetite,* 1993. 21(3): 247–54.

Lazar, S. W., et al. Functional brain mapping of the relaxation response and meditation. *Neuroreport,* 2000. 11(7): 1581–85.

Leventhal, L., et al. Selective actions of central mu and kappa opioid antagonists upon sucrose intake in sham-fed rats. *Brain Res,* 1995. 685(1–2): 205–10.

Levine, A. S., C. M. Kotz, and B. A. Gosnell. Sugars: hedonic aspects, neuroregulation, and energy balance. *Am J Clin Nutr,* 2003. 78(4): 834S–42S.

———. Sugars and fats: the neurobiology of preference. *J Nutr,* 2003. 133(3): 831S–34S.

Levine, A. S., et al. Opioids and consummatory behavior. *Brain Res Bull,* 1985. 14(6): 663–72.

Levine, A. S., et al. Neuropeptides as regulators of consummatory behaviors. *J Nutr,* 1986. 116(11): 2067–77.

Lewis, M. E., et al. Opiate receptor localization in rat cerebral cortex. *J Comp Neurol,* 1983. 216(3): 339–58.

Lieblich, I., et al. Morphine tolerance in genetically selected rats induced by chronically elevated saccharin intake. *Science,* 1983. 221(4613): 871–73.

Lovell, H. W., and J. W. Tintera. Hypoadrenocorticism in alcoholism and drug addiction. *Geriatrics,* 1951. 6(1): 1–11.

Macdiarmid, J. I., and M. M. Hetherington. Mood modulation by food: an exploration of affect and cravings in "chocolate addicts." *Br J Clin Psychol,* 1995. 34 (Pt 1): 129–38.

Mahoney, C. R., et al. Effect of breakfast composition on cognitive processes in elementary school children. *Physiol Behav*, 2005. 85(5): 635–45.

Marinelli, P. W., R. Quirion, and C. Gianoulakis. An in vivo profile of beta-endorphin release in the arcuate nucleus and nucleus accumbens following exposure to stress or alcohol. *Neuroscience*, 2004. 127(3): 777–84.

Markovitz, D. C., and J. D. Fernstrom, Diet and uptake of aldomet by the brain: competition with natural large neutral amino acids. *Science*, 1977. 197(4307): 1014–15.

Mathes, W. F., and R. B. Kanarek. Wheel running attenuates the antinociceptive properties of morphine and its metabolite, morphine-6-glucuronide, in rats. *Physiol Behav*, 2001. 74(1–2): 245–51.

Mitchell, J. E., et al. The relationship between compulsive buying and eating disorders. *Int J Eat Disord*, 2002. 32(1): 107–11.

Moles, A., and S. J. Cooper. Opioid modulation of sucrose intake in CD-1 mice: effects of gender and housing conditions. *Physiol Behav*, 1995. 58(4): 791–96.

Morley, J. E., et al. Which opioid receptor mechanism modulates feeding? *Appetite*, 1984. 5(1): 61–68.

Niesink, R. J., L. J. Vanderschuren, and J. M. van Ree. Social play in juvenile rats after in utero exposure to morphine. *Neurotoxicology*, 1996. 17(3–4): 905–12.

Pert, C. B., M. J. Kuhar, and S. H. Snyder. Autoradiographic localization of the opiate receptor in rat brain. *Life Sci*, 1975. 16(12): 1849–53.

Putzke, J., et al. Long-term alcohol self-administration and alcohol withdrawal differentially modulate microtubule-associated protein 2 (MAP2) gene expression in the rat brain. *Brain Res Mol Brain Res*, 1998. 62(2): 196–205.

Rada, P., N. M. Avena, and B. G. Hoebel. Daily bingeing on sugar repeatedly releases dopamine in the accumbens shell. *Neuroscience*, 2005. 134(3): 737–44.

Rakatansky, H. Chocolate: pleasure or pain? *R I Med*, 1995. 78(7): 179.

Reid, L. D., et al. Opioids and intake of alcoholic beverages. *NIDA Res Monogr*, 1986. 75: 359–62.

Ripsin, C. M., et al. Oat products and lipid lowering. A meta-analysis. *JAMA*, 1992. 267(24): 3317–25.

Roach, M. K., and R. J. Williams. Impaired and inadequate glucose metabolism in the brain as an underlying cause of alcoholism—an hypothesis. *Proc Natl Acad Sci USA*, 1966. 56(2): 566–71.

Ruegg, H., W. Z. Yu, and R. J. Bodnar. Opioid-receptor subtype agonist-induced enhancements of sucrose intake are dependent upon sucrose concentration. *Physiol Behav*, 1997. 62(1): 121–28.

Sato, Y., et al. Improved insulin sensitivity in carbohydrate and lipid metabolism after physical training. *Int J Sports Med*, 1986. 7(6): 307–10.

Schoenbaum, G. M., R. J. Martin, and D. S. Roane. Relationships between sustained sucrose-feeding and opioid tolerance and withdrawal. *Pharmacol Biochem Behav*, 1989. 34(4): 911–14.

Segato, F. N., et al. Sucrose ingestion causes opioid analgesia. *Braz J Med Biol Res*, 1997. 30(8): 981–84.

Semenova, S., A. Kuzmin, and E. Zvartau. Strain differences in the analgesic and reinforcing action of morphine in mice. *Pharmacol Biochem Behav*, 1995. 50(1): 17–21.

Sforzo, G. A., et al. In vivo opioid receptor occupation in the rat brain following exercise. *Med Sci Sports Exerc*, 1986. 18(4): 380–84.

Shide, D. J., and E. M. Blass. Opioid mediation of odor preferences induced by sugar and fat in 6-day-old rats. *Physiol Behav*, 1991. 50(5): 961–66.

Shippenberg, T. S., et al. Conditioning of opioid reinforcement: neuroanatomical and neurochemical substrates. *Ann N Y Acad Sci*, 1992. 654: 347–56.

Shoemaker, W. J., and P. Kehoe. Effect of isolation conditions on brain regional enkephalin and beta-endorphin levels and vocalizations in 10-day-old rat pups. *Behav Neurosci*, 1995. 109(1): 117–22.

Sillaber, I., et al. Enhanced morphine-induced behavioural effects and dopamine release in the nucleus accumbens in a transgenic mouse model of impaired glucocorticoid (type II) receptor function: influence of long-term treatment with the antidepressant moclobemide. *Neuroscience*, 1998. 85(2): 415–25.

Sipols, A. J., et al. Intraventricular insulin decreases kappa opioid-mediated sucrose intake in rats. *Peptides*, 2002. 23(12): 2181–87.

Snyder, S. H., and R. Simantov. The opiate receptor and opioid peptides. *J Neurochem*, 1977. 28(1): 13–20.

Spanagel, R. The influence of opioid antagonists on the discriminative stimulus effects of ethanol. *Pharmacol Biochem Behav*, 1996. 54(4): 645–49.

Spanagel, R., and M. Heilig. Addiction and its brain science. *Addiction*, 2005. 100(12): 1813–22.

Spanagel, R., O. F. Almeida, and T. S. Shippenberg. Long lasting changes in morphine-induced mesolimbic dopamine release after chronic morphine exposure. *Synapse*, 1993. 14(3): 243–45.

Spanagel, R., A. Herz, and T. S. Shippenberg. The effects of opioid peptides on dopamine release in the nucleus accumbens: an in vivo microdialysis study. *J Neurochem*, 1990. 55(5): 1734–40.

Spanagel, R., et al. Beta-endorphin-induced locomotor stimulation and reinforcement are associated with an increase in dopamine release in the nucleus accumbens. *Psychopharmacology* (Berl), 1991. 104(1): 51–56.

Spanagel, R., et al. Endogenous kappa-opioid systems in opiate withdrawal: role in aversion and accompanying changes in mesolimbic dopamine release. *Psychopharmacology* (Berl), 1994. 115(1–2): 121–27.

Spangler, R., et al. Elevated D3 dopamine receptor mRNA in dopaminergic and dopaminoceptive regions of the rat brain in response to morphine. *Brain Res Mol Brain Res*, 2003. 111(1–2): 74–83.

Spangler, R., et al. Opiate-like effects of sugar on gene expression in reward areas of the rat brain. *Brain Res Mol Brain Res*, 2004. 124(2): 134–42.

van der Kolk, B. A. The body keeps the score: memory and the evolving psychobiology of posttraumatic stress. *Harv Rev Psychiatry*, 1994. 1(5): 253–65.

———. Clinical implications of neuroscience research in PTSD. *Ann N Y Acad Sci*, 2006. 1071: 277–93.

van der Kolk, B. A., et al. Disorders of extreme stress: the empirical foundation of a complex adaptation to trauma. *J Trauma Stress*, 2005. 18(5): 389–99.

van Gaalen, M. M., et al. Critical involvement of dopaminergic neurotransmission in impulsive decision making. *Biol Psychiatry*, 2006. 60(1): 66–73.

van Ree, J. M., et al. Endogenous opioids and reward. *Eur J Pharmacol*, 2000. 405(1–3): 89–101.

van Wymelbeke, V., et al. Influence of repeated consumption of beverages containing sucrose or intense sweeteners on food intake. *Eur J Clin Nutr*, 2004. 58(1): 154–61.

Vanderschuren, L. J., et al. A single exposure to morphine induces long-lasting behavioural and neurochemical sensitization in rats. *Eur J Neurosci*, 2001. 14(9): 1533–38.

Vanderschuren, L. J., et al. Morphine-induced long-term sensitization to the locomotor effects of morphine and amphetamine depends on the temporal pattern of the pretreatment regimen. *Psychopharmacology* (Berl), 1997. 131(2): 115–22.

Vaughan, C. W., et al. Cellular actions of opioids on periaqueductal grey neurons from C57B16/J mice and mutant mice lacking MOR-1. *Br J Pharmacol*, 2003. 139(2): 362–67.

Wideman, C. H., G. R. Nadzam, and H. M. Murphy. Implications of an animal model of sugar addiction, withdrawal and relapse for human health. *Nutr Neurosci*, 2005. 8(5–6): 269–76.

Williams, R. J. Alcoholism as a nutritional problem. *Am J Clin Nutr*, 1952. 1(1): 32–36.

———. Biochemical individuality and cellular nutrition: prime factors in alcoholism. *Q J Stud Alcohol*, 1959. 20: 452–63.

Williams, R. J., L. J. Berry, and E. Beerstecher. Individual metabolic patterns, alcoholism, genetotrophic diseases. *Proc Natl Acad Sci USA*, 1949. 35(6): 265–71.

Wurtman, R. J., and J. J. Wurtman. Brain serotonin, carbohydrate-craving, obesity and depression. *Adv Exp Med Biol*, 1996. 398: 35–41.

RESOURCES

WEBSITE

Find Radiant Recovery® on the web at **www.radiantrecovery**
.com or email us at **admin@radiantrecovery.com**. We are always
delighted to have your feedback and comments. You will find a
wide variety of tools on the site to support you in doing the program. Be sure to sign up for our weekly newsletter and to click on
the link "Getting Started."

NEWSLETTER

We send out a weekly newsletter free of charge. It's not just fluff.
You'll find information on new classes, personal stories by our
members, reports from the various online support groups, and
articles by Kathleen. Come to the website to sign up.

GEORGE'S® SHAKE

Our shake mix is the cornerstone of the program for many of our
community members. We now have three varieties of the famous
George's® Shake.

- *George's® Original* contains a mixture of proteins, a complex carb, and all your daily vitamins all in one package. The primary protein is soy, which makes it ideal for older women.
- *George's® Restore* is a whey protein isolate formula with incomparable taste. It is perfect for those who prefer a nonsoy formula or who wish to increase the protein in the shake without adding more vitamins. It is also perfect for pregnant and breastfeeding women. It is very easy to mix so it is great for traveling.
- *George's® Junior* is a special formula for children and teens. It has a very mild taste that mixes well with all flavorings.

We also carry a wide variety of flavorings to add to your shake. Check our store at **www.radiantrecoverystore.com.**

MOTIVATIONAL TOOLS
Books

Here are the other books Kathleen has written since the first publication of *Potatoes Not Prozac.*

- *The Sugar Addict's Total Recovery Program* is a great how-to manual on doing the program day to day. It also has some wonderful recipes.
- *Your Last Diet!* is our weight-loss bible.
- *Little Sugar Addicts* is a wonderful guide for sugar-sensitive parents wanting to help their sugar-sensitive children.
- *Your Body Speaks* is the food journal we created especially for sugar-sensitive people.
- *Radiant Recipes* is our very own cookbook of yummy but program-friendly foods created by Kathleen and a personal chef.
- *The DUI Diet* is Kathleen's Ph.D. dissertation on how she achieved an unheard-of 92 percent success rate using her

food plan for sugar sensitivity to help multiple-offender drunk drivers stop drinking.

Audio

Potatoes Not Prozac (the first edition) and *The Sugar Addict's Total Recovery Program* are both available on CD. We also have a variety of other audio programs by Kathleen to help support your program, including:

- *Introduction to the Biochemistry of Sugar Sensitivity* (CD)
- *The Warrior Spirit: How Your Attitude Shapes Your Program* (CD)
- *Successfully Parenting a Sugar-Sensitive Child* (CD)
- *What Else Is Embedded in the Steps* (CD)
- *Radiant Ranch 2007*

Support Groups

We have online support groups for each step in the program and for anyone with a special situation. For example, there are groups for diabetics, people with more than one hundred pounds to lose, men, parents of sugar-sensitive children; for fitness; for people who are just starting to exercise; for people with eating disorders, depression; and even pets. We also offer support groups for all the regions of the United States, Europe, and Australia. Go to **www .radiantrecovery.com** and click on the "Make Connections" link to find a group that suits your needs.

Weight Loss

We provide an online weight loss program specifically designed for sugar-sensitive people called "Your Last Diet Online." It includes classes, special online support groups, live online chats with Kathleen, and many other resources for successful weight loss.

Seminars

Kathleen leads seminars regularly throughout the United States and Europe. Check the website or call the office at 888-579-3970 for more information.

Online Classes

Our low-cost online classes cover a wide variety of topics, including how to do each individual step in the program, brain chemistry (serotonin, beta-endorphin, and dopamine), what to do at holidays, how to lose weight, special issues for parents, and other concerns like depression, anxiety, IBD, and diabetes.

Consulting with Kathleen

Kathleen does telephone consultation with people from all over the world. Check the website under "Make Connections" for more information.

Radiant Recovery® Store

The online store at **www.radiantrecoverystore.com** is the hub for sales of all our products. Kathleen personally reviews and selects all the items we carry.

INDEX